BREAKTHROUGH SERIES Guide

MW01049268

Reducing Delays and Waiting Times Throughout the Healthcare System

Thomas W. Nolan

Marie W. Schall

Donald M. Berwick

Jane Roessner

INSTITUTE FOR HEALTHCARE IMPROVEMENT

Institute for Healthcare Improvement
135 Francis Street
Boston, MA 02215
(617) 754-4800

Breakthrough Series Guides
Managing Editor: Penny Carver, MEd
Design and Composition:
Matt Kanaracus, Karen LeDuc

Guide to Reducing Delays and Waiting Times
Authors: Thomas W. Nolan, PhD
Marie W. Schall, MA
Donald M. Berwick, MD
Jane Roessner, PhD

First Edition
Printed in the USA
10 9 8 7 6 5 4

Library of Congress Catalog
Card Number: 96-79933

ISBN 1-890070-00-9

INSTITUTE FOR HEALTHCARE IMPROVEMENT

The Institute for Healthcare Improvement (IHI) is a nonprofit organization designed to be a major force for integrative and collaborative efforts to accelerate improvement in the healthcare systems of the United States and Canada. The Institute provides bridges connecting people and organizations who are committed to real reforms, and who believe that they can accomplish more together than they can separately.

In addition to the Breakthrough Series, IHI offers courses, the annual National Forum on Quality Improvement in Health Care, networks of healthcare organizations engaged in change, and research and demonstration projects in regulation and professional education reform.

For more information about the Breakthrough Series activities and publications, as well as other programs and activities sponsored by the Institute for Healthcare Improvement, please call (617) 754-4800, fax (617) 754-4848 or write to IHI, 135 Francis Street, Boston, MA 02215.

ABOUT THE BREAKTHROUGH SERIES

The Breakthrough Series was developed by the Institute for Healthcare Improvement to bring together groups of healthcare organizations that share a commitment to making major, rapid changes that will produce breakthrough results: lower cost and better outcomes at the same time.

Each collaborative in the Breakthrough Series includes 20 to 40 healthcare organizations focusing on a single topic—gathering and studying the latest scientific information available on improving specific clinical or operational areas, and learning effective means to put that knowledge into practice for rapid improvement.

Breakthrough Series topics are chosen because they are "ripe" for improvement:

- Substantial knowledge exists about how to achieve better performance.
- There is a gap between the best available knowledge and actual everyday practice.
- Strong examples already exist of organizations (even if only a few) that have applied that knowledge and "broken through" to unprecedented results.
- Improvement is responsive to demands for health care that is both lower in cost and able to achieve better clinical outcomes with much higher satisfaction for all who depend on the healthcare system.

BREAKTHROUGH SERIES TOPICS

Reducing Delays and Waiting Times Throughout the Healthcare System

Reducing Cesarean Section Rates While Maintaining Maternal and Infant Outcomes

Improving Asthma Care in Children and Adults

Reducing Adverse Drug Events and Medical Errors

Reducing Costs and Improving Outcomes in Adult Intensive Care

Reducing Costs and Improving Outcomes in Adult Cardiac Surgery

Providing More Effective Care for Low Back Pain

Improving Inpatient and Outpatient Physician Prescribing Practices

Reducing Costs and Improving Outcomes in Neonatal Intensive Care

Improving Inventory Levels and Supplier Management

Improving Care of the Dying

Reducing Costs While Improving Quality Throughout the Healthcare System

BREAKTHROUGH SERIES COLLABORATIVE ON REDUCING DELAYS AND WAITING TIMES

PLANNING GROUP

The Institute for Healthcare Improvement wishes to thank our Collaborative Chair and Director and the members of the Planning Group for their dedication, wit, and wisdom. They share a vision of a healthcare system that keeps no one waiting—patient, family, nurse, physician—and a determination to make that vision a reality.

Thomas Nolan, PhD
Statistician
Associates in Process Improvement
Silver Springs, MD
Collaborative Chair

Marie W. Schall, MA
Institute for Healthcare Improvement
Boston, MA
Collaborative Director

G. Ross Baker, PhD
Department of Health Administration
University of Toronto
Toronto, ON

Sherry Delio, MPA, HSA
Director of Practice Administration
Mercy Integrated Health System
Phoenix, AZ

Charles M. Kilo, MD, MPH
Institute for Healthcare Improvement
Boston, MA

Jean Krause, BS, RRA
Director, Quality Improvement
Franciscan Skemp Healthcare–Mayo
Health System
La Crosse, WI

Robert Lederer, MD
Assistant to Medical Director,
Best Practices
Kaiser Permanente Colorado
Denver, CO

Sharon Linton, MBA
Manager, Customer Satisfaction Education
Eddie Bauer, Inc.
Bellevue, WA

Linda J. Mild, RN, MS
Senior Vice President, Clinical Services
Columbia Wesley Medical Center
Wichita, KS

Patricia A. Rutherford, RN, MS
Nursing/Patient Services Director
Children's Hospital
Boston, MA

The Breakthrough Series Guides are designed for healthcare practitioners who want to make change.

When do you need a guidebook? When you want to go somewhere you've never been before, or learn how to do something you've never done before. Guidebooks can also be useful when you're returning to a place you have visited before. Whether you are new to reducing delays or returning to the effort, you will profit from this guide.

What do you need in a guide? Clear explanations, useful tips, and step-by-step instruction—so that you can learn as quickly as possible. Practical and user-friendly, the Breakthrough Series Guides are based on the real experiences of healthcare organizations that have made change. The aim of the Guides is to disseminate what the collaborative organizations have learned as widely as possible, in order to help others design and implement their own breakthrough improvements.

Contents

	Acknowledgments	xii
	Introduction	xiv
	The Challenge, the Goal, the Results	
Part 1	**A Model for Accelerating Improvement**	1
Part 2	**A Step-by-Step Guide to Reducing Delays and Waiting Times**	11
	Setting Aims	12
	Forming the Team	16
	Establishing Measures	20
	Developing and Testing Changes	24
Part 3	**27 Change Concepts for Reducing Delays and Waiting Times**	31
	Redesigning the System	42
	Shaping Demand	54
	Matching Capacity to Demand	64
Part 4	**Achieving Breakthrough Improvement in Four Key Areas**	73
	Reducing Delays in Surgery	76
	Reducing Delays in the Emergency Department	92
	Reducing Waiting Times in Clinics and Physicians' Offices	108
	Increasing Access to Care	122
Part 5	**Troubleshooting: Overcoming Barriers to Change**	137
Part 6	**Resources for Reducing Delays and Waiting Times**	149
	Breakthrough Series Assessment	150
	Summary of Aims, Changes and Results	152
	Key Contacts	168
	Quality Improvement Storyboards	172
	Improvement Cycle Worksheet	178
	Annotated Bibliography	180

THANKS

Thanks to all of the organizations that took part in the Breakthrough Series Collaborative on Reducing Delays and Waiting Times. They made a commitment to making major, rapid changes in their organizations. They are the true guides; they generously shared their insights, their successes, and the lessons they learned along the way—and in so doing, they have paved the way for others to follow.

Beth Israel Deaconess Medical Center–
East Campus
Boston, MA

Beth Israel Deaconess Medical Center–
West Campus
Boston, MA

Cambridge Hospital
Cambridge, MA

Chester County Hospital
West Chester, PA

Children's Hospital
Boston, MA

Christ Hospital
Jersey City, NJ

Columbia Wesley Medical Center
Wichita, KS

Covenant Healthcare System, Inc.
Milwaukee, WI

Dartmouth-Hitchcock Medical Center
Lebanon, NH

Deborah Heart and Lung Center
Browns Mills, NJ

Department of Veterans Affairs
Medical Center
New Orleans, LA

Franciscan Skemp Healthcare–
Mayo Health System
La Crosse, WI

GHMA Medical Centers/HealthPartners
of Southern Arizona
Tucson, AZ

Glens Falls Hospital
Glens Falls, NY

Group Health Cooperative of Puget
Sound
Tacoma, WA

HealthPartners
Minneapolis, MN

HealthSystem Minnesota
St. Louis Park, MN

Kaiser Permanente Colorado
Denver, CO

MetroHealth
Indianapolis, IN

Northwest Covenant Medical Center
Denville, NJ

Sewickley Valley Hospital
Sewickley, PA

SSM Health Care System
St. Louis, MO

SSM Health Care System/
St. Francis Hospital & Health Center
Blue Island, IL

SSM Health Care System/
St. Mary's Health Center
St. Louis, MO

St. Joseph's Mercy Hospitals
and Health Services
Clinton Township, MI

UNITY Choice Health Plan
Des Moines, IA

University of Michigan Medical Center
Ann Arbor, MI

VHA Pennsylvania, Inc.
Pittsburgh, PA

Virginia Mason Medical Center
Seattle, WA

Watson Clinic LLP
Lakeland, FL

York Health System
York, PA

Introduction The Challenge

Significant reductions in delays and waiting times are possible.

Increasing access to care—without adding staff—is possible.

How? By redesigning the system.

"Toyota revolutionized our expectations of production; Federal Express revolutionized our expectations of service. Processes that once took days or hours to complete are now measured in minutes or seconds. The challenge is to revolutionize our expectations of health care: to design a continuous flow of work for clinicians and a seamless experience of care for patients."

Donald M. Berwick, MD
President and CEO, Institute for Healthcare Improvement

The healthcare system is currently designed to produce exactly the levels of delays and access we now experience. Results, costs, waiting times, access to services—all are properties of the system of work itself. Performance is not simply—it is not even mainly—a matter of effort; it is a matter of design.

Therefore, if we want to reduce delays and increase access, we need to redesign the system that produces them. Better results, lower costs, shorter waiting times, increased access—these will only be achieved by changing the way we do our work.

Reduced delays and increased access are among the most important dimensions on which healthcare systems will be judged over the coming years. As large payers drive prices lower, competition among healthcare organizations is shifting to service and quality. Organizations that are able to respond to their customers' expectations of timely access to care will have the competitive advantage.

"People often assume that reducing delays and increasing access will increase cost. In fact, the opposite is true: delays and restricted access are properties of poorly designed, costly systems. The same changes that reduce delays and increase access can also reduce cost."

Thomas W. Nolan, PhD
Statistician, Associates in Process Improvement

Indeed, some managed care contracts now set targets for reducing delays and increasing access—getting an appointment within seven days, waiting no more than 10 minutes. One way healthcare organizations can meet these targets is to add more providers; another way is to redesign the system without increasing resources.

The true costs of delays—and thus, the opportunities for improvement—are several. Consider the following:

- The patient waiting to be transferred from the ICU to a patient care unit is not just a service issue; the ICU is a very expensive place to wait.
- The clinic that must meet a target of offering appointments within seven days has two choices: hire more physicians and staff, or redesign the system to meet the target without any new hiring.
- The hospital that can reduce the time it takes to do surgery by 25% has just significantly increased the capacity of its OR and staff.

The Goal

In June 1995, 27 healthcare organizations began working together to reduce delays and waiting times, and increase access to care, as part of the Institute for Healthcare Improvement's Breakthrough Series. Their goal: 50% reduction in delays and waiting times within 12 months.

Although the goal was ambitious, the participants felt that it was both reasonable and achievable, based on evidence that at least 50% of the total duration of most care processes consisted of waiting time. Moreover, the goal conveyed a clear message: small, incremental changes would not be enough; only large, breakthrough changes would lead to the goal.

Note: For a complete summary of the Collaborative organizations' aims, major changes and results, see Part 6.

Figure 0.1

MEDIAN DELAY IN SURGERY: 11 AM AND 2 PM

Sewickley Valley Hospital
Sewickley, PA

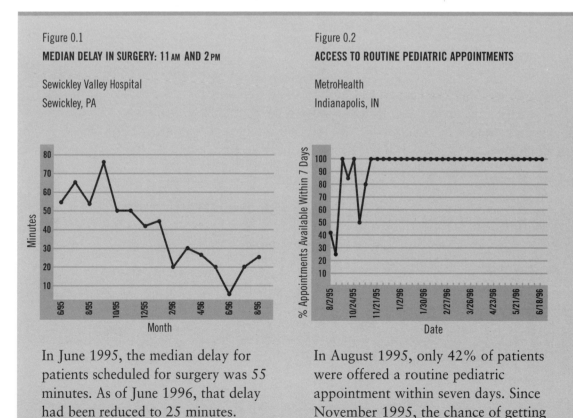

In June 1995, the median delay for patients scheduled for surgery was 55 minutes. As of June 1996, that delay had been reduced to 25 minutes.

Figure 0.2

ACCESS TO ROUTINE PEDIATRIC APPOINTMENTS

MetroHealth
Indianapolis, IN

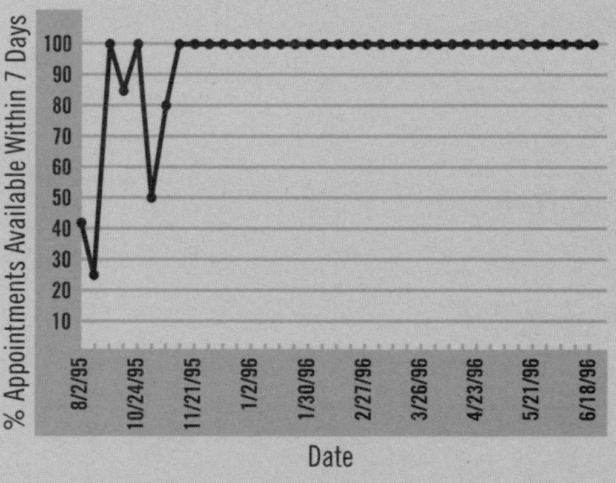

In August 1995, only 42% of patients were offered a routine pediatric appointment within seven days. Since November 1995, the chance of getting the appointment within seven days has been 100%.

The Results

Many organizations met and exceeded their initial goal of 50% reduction in delays and waiting times. Others, while still short of their goal, made substantial progress.

The four examples below are illustrative of the significant reductions in delays and waiting times—in surgery, emergency department, clinics and physicians' offices, and access to care—achieved by organizations in the Breakthrough Series over 12 months.

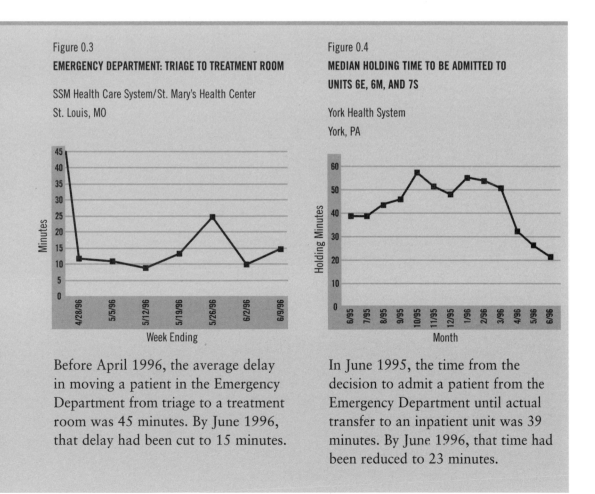

Figure 0.3

EMERGENCY DEPARTMENT: TRIAGE TO TREATMENT ROOM

SSM Health Care System/St. Mary's Health Center
St. Louis, MO

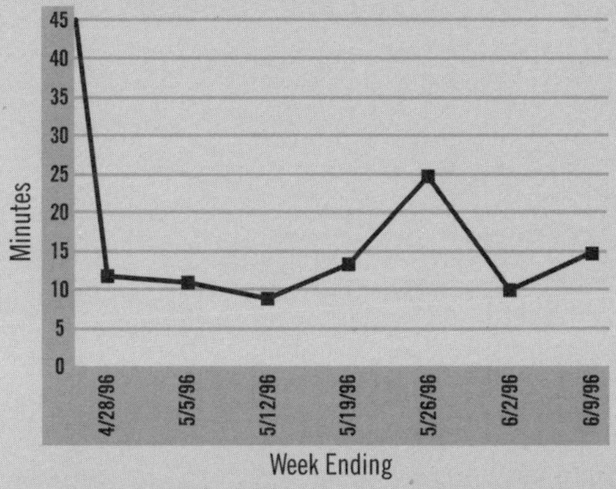

Before April 1996, the average delay in moving a patient in the Emergency Department from triage to a treatment room was 45 minutes. By June 1996, that delay had been cut to 15 minutes.

Figure 0.4

MEDIAN HOLDING TIME TO BE ADMITTED TO UNITS 6E, 6M, AND 7S

York Health System
York, PA

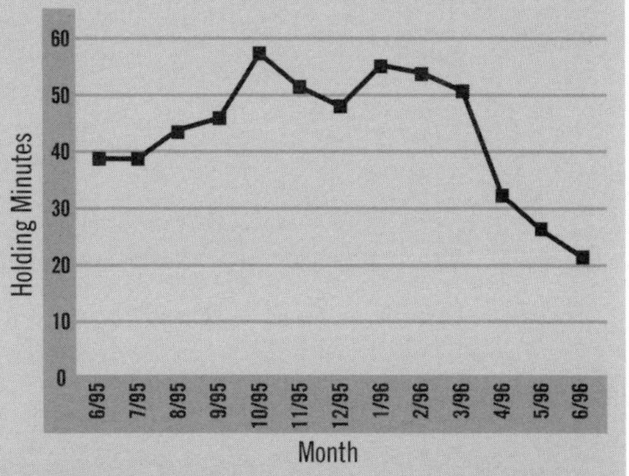

In June 1995, the time from the decision to admit a patient from the Emergency Department until actual transfer to an inpatient unit was 39 minutes. By June 1996, that time had been reduced to 23 minutes.

Part 1

A Model for Accelerating Improvement

This section introduces the Model for Improvement and shows how one organization used the model to reduce delays in its Emergency Department.

The Model for Improvement

Organizations in the Breakthrough Series use a simple yet powerful model for improvement. The model is not meant to replace change models that organizations may already be using, but rather to accelerate improvement.

The model has two parts:

- Three fundamental questions, which can be addressed in any order.
- The Plan-Do-Study-Act (PDSA) cycle to test and implement changes in real work settings.

The Model for Improvement was initially developed by Tom Nolan and colleagues at Associates in Process Improvement, as a framework for accelerating improvement in a variety of business contexts (see Langley G, Nolan K, Nolan T, Norman C, Provost L. *The Improvement Guide: A Practical Approach to Enhancing Organizational Performance.* San Francisco: Jossey-Bass Publishers; 1996).

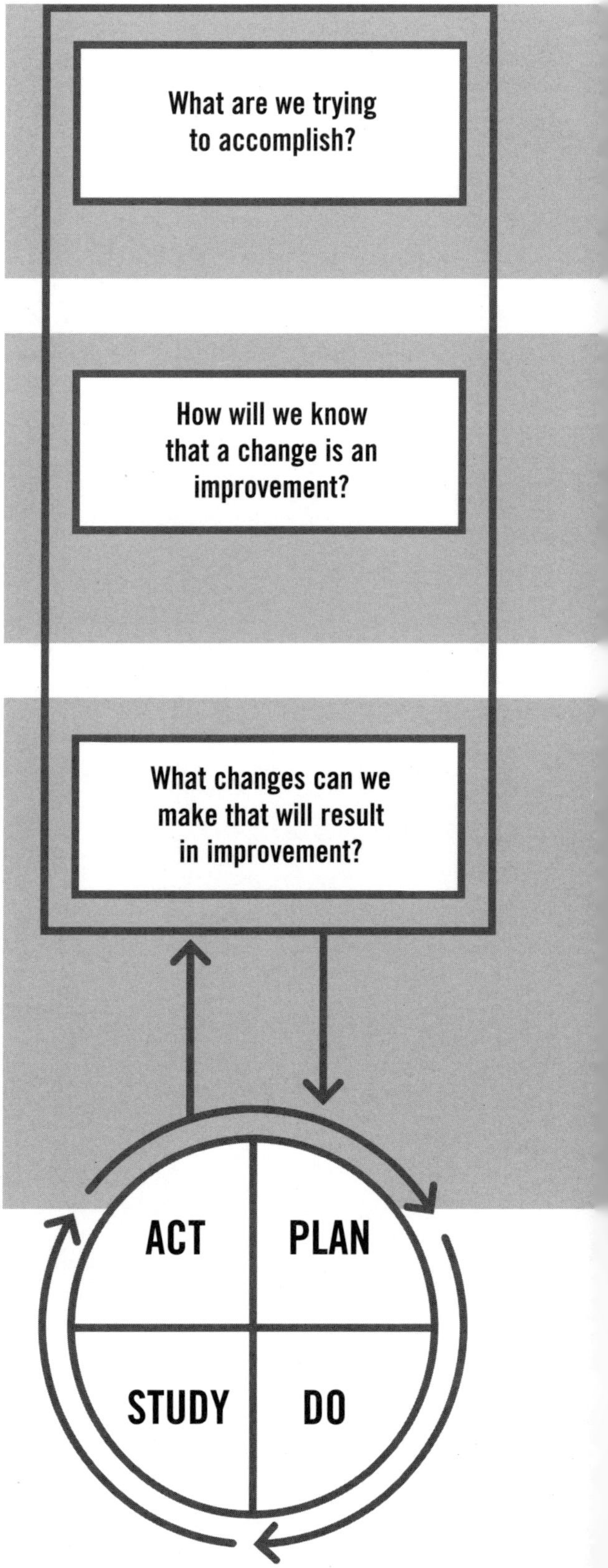

SETTING AIMS

Improvement begins with setting aims. An organization will not improve without a clear and firm intention to do so. Moreover, the aim should be expressed in specific terms—e.g., 50% reduction in delays in surgery, 30% reduction in cesarean section rates, 50% reduction in adverse drug events. Agreement on the aim is crucial, as is allocation of the people and resources necessary to accomplish the aim.

ESTABLISHING MEASURES

Measurement is an important part of testing and implementing changes. Measures need to be identified to indicate whether a change that is made actually leads to an improvement. Measures are used for learning (e.g., Were delays in surgery reduced after all key surgical processes were synchronized around the point of incision? Were delays in the ED reduced after a separate process was created to treat nonemergent cases? Were additional same-day appointments available after the scheduling system was simplified?).

DEVELOPING CHANGES

All improvement requires making a change, but not all changes result in improvement. Since achieving new goals requires changing the system, it is important to be able to identify the most promising changes.

Many sources can contribute good ideas for changes: critical thinking about the current system, creative thinking, watching the process, a hunch, getting insight from a completely different situation, and more. This Guide refers to good, general ideas for change as "change concepts." A change concept is a general idea—with proven merit and a sound scientific or logical foundation—that can stimulate specific ideas for changes that lead to improvement. Using change concepts, and combining them creatively, can stimulate new ways of thinking about the problem at hand.

For a comprehensive list of ideas for change that can help reduce delays in any system, see Part 3, 27 Change Concepts for Reducing Delays and Waiting Times.

TESTING CHANGES

Once a team has set an aim, established measures to indicate whether a change leads to an improvement, and found a promising idea for change, the next step is to test that change in the real work setting by conducting a Plan-Do-Study-Act (PDSA) cycle.

THE PLAN-DO-STUDY-ACT CYCLE

The Model for Improvement is based on a "trial-and-learning" approach to improvement. The PDSA cycle describes how to test a change—by trying it, observing the consequences, and then learning from those consequences.

Several challenges need to be addressed in each step of the PDSA cycle:

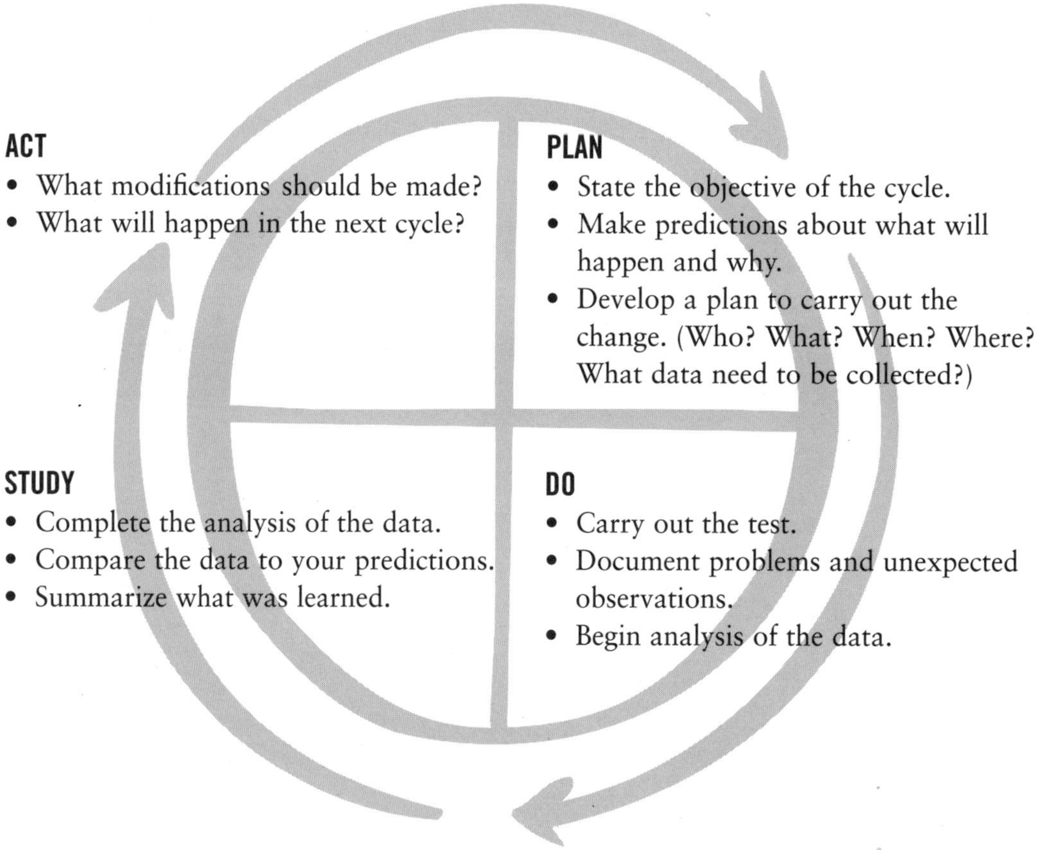
ACT
• What modifications should be made?
• What will happen in the next cycle?
PLAN
• State the objective of the cycle.
• Make predictions about what will happen and why.
• Develop a plan to carry out the change. (Who? What? When? Where? What data need to be collected?)
STUDY
• Complete the analysis of the data.
• Compare the data to your predictions.
• Summarize what was learned.
DO
• Carry out the test.
• Document problems and unexpected observations.
• Begin analysis of the data.

Note: For a detailed example documenting a PDSA cycle, see the Improvement Cycle Worksheet in Part 6, Resources for Reducing Delays and Waiting Times.

It is often better to run small cycles soon rather than large cycles later, after a long period of planning. The change may be very ambitious and innovative, but it should be tested on a small scale—for example, with only one or two physicians, in one or two operating rooms, or with the next three patients. Each PDSA cycle, properly done, is informative and provides a basis for further improvement. Once you know that a change works and you have been able to improve it over several PDSA cycles, then you can implement it on a larger scale.

LINKING PLAN-DO-STUDY-ACT CYCLES INTO RAMPS

The completion of each PDSA cycle leads directly into the start of the next cycle. A team learns from the test (What worked and what didn't work? What should be kept, changed or thrown out?) and uses the new knowledge to plan the next test. The team continues linking PDSA cycles in this way until the change is ready for broader implementation. These linked PDSA cycles are called "ramps."

People are far more willing to test a change if they know that changes can and will be amended as necessary. Linking small cycles in this way helps overcome an organization's natural resistance to change.

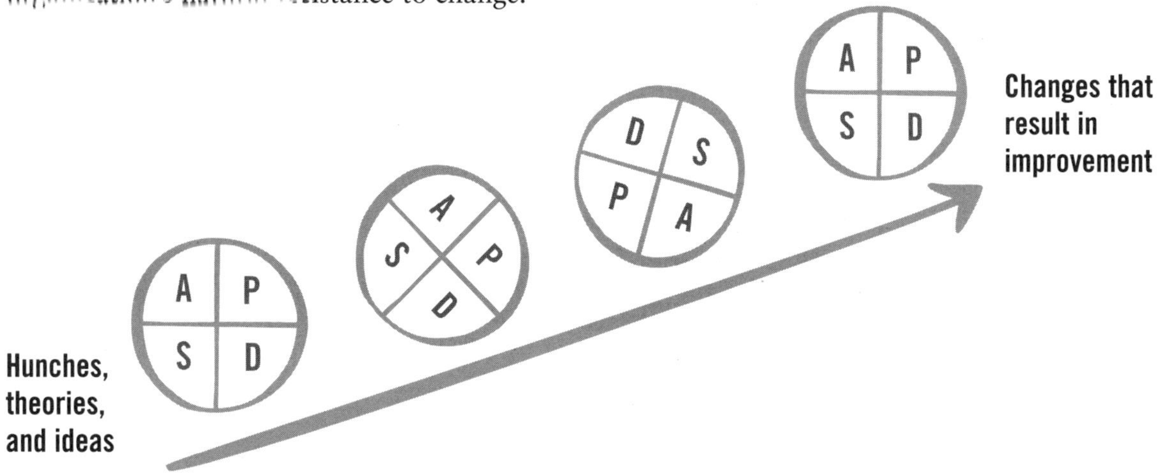

MULTIPLE RAMPS

Often, teams are involved in testing more than one change at a time. The linked tests for each change form a ramp; when a team is testing several different changes, it will have several different ramps.

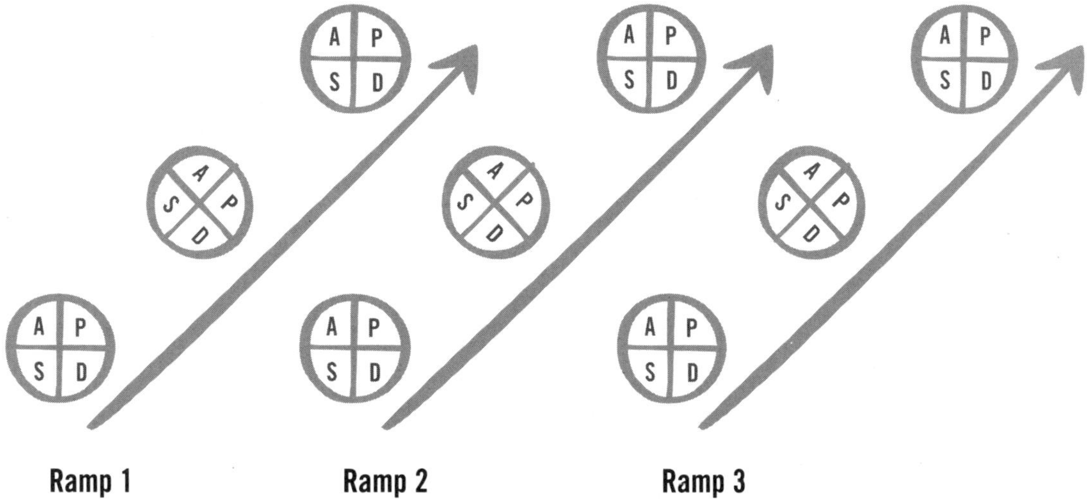

Case Study: York Health System

York Health System's 558-bed community teaching hospital was experiencing delays in moving patients from the Emergency Department into inpatient beds. The ED was in effect becoming a holding area for patients who needed beds.

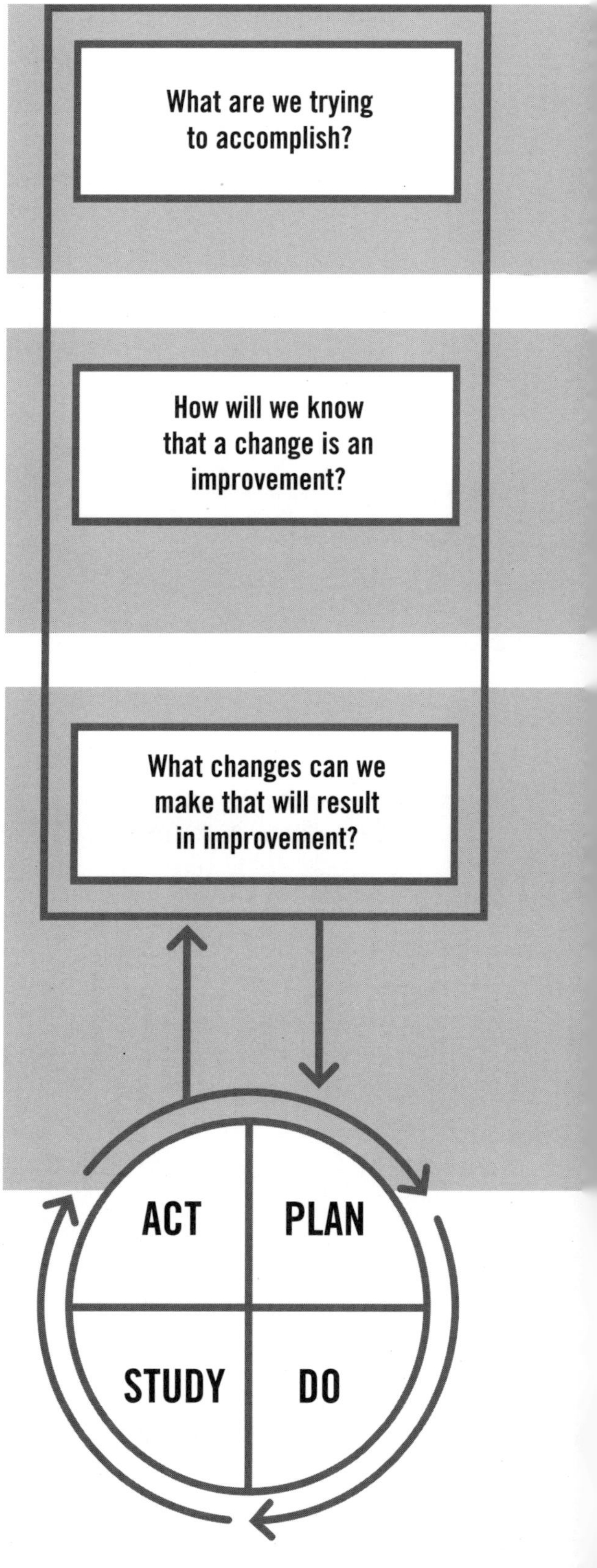

SETTING AIMS

The team set the following aim: Reduce delays in transferring patients from the Emergency Department to inpatient beds by 50%.

ESTABLISHING MEASURES

The team established the following measure: A change is an improvement if the time it takes to transfer a patient from the Emergency Department (ED) to an inpatient unit decreases.

The team measured the time from when a decision was made to admit a patient from the ED until the time the patient was actually taken to the unit.

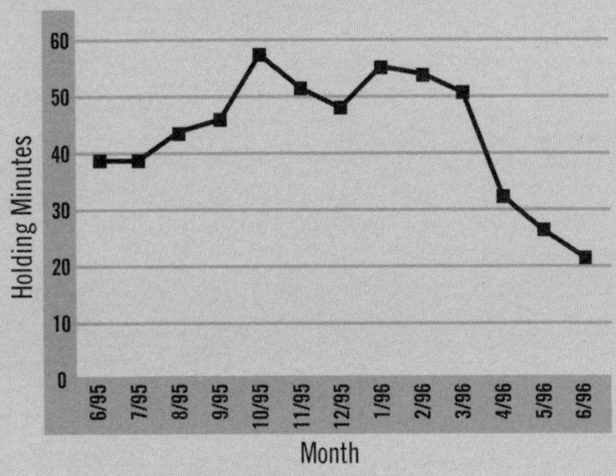

Figure 1.1
MEDIAN HOLDING TIME TO BE ADMITTED TO UNITS 6E, 6M, AND 7S

York Health System
York, PA

DEVELOPING CHANGES

In order to find good ideas for changes, the team began by examining the existing process. Team members found that delays in the transfer of patients from the ED were occurring because there were no beds available in the ICU. In order to reduce ED delays, changes would have to be made to free up beds in the ICU.

TESTING CHANGES

The team's first "hunch" was that improved utilization of intensive care, transitional, and telemetry beds would result in reduced delays for patients in the ED.

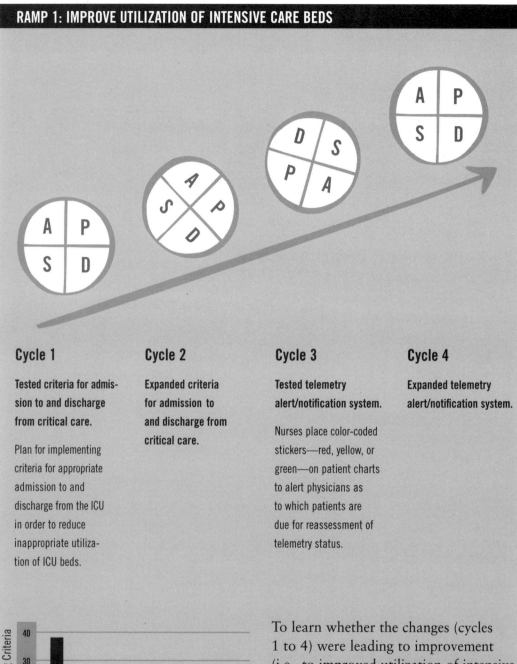

RAMP 1: IMPROVE UTILIZATION OF INTENSIVE CARE BEDS

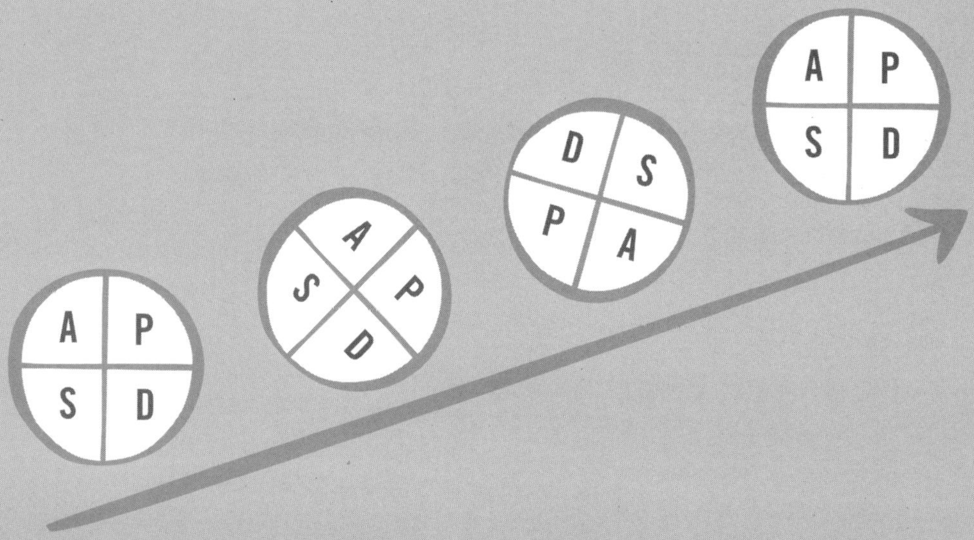

Cycle 1

Tested criteria for admission to and discharge from critical care.

Plan for implementing criteria for appropriate admission to and discharge from the ICU in order to reduce inappropriate utilization of ICU beds.

Cycle 2

Expanded criteria for admission to and discharge from critical care.

Cycle 3

Tested telemetry alert/notification system.

Nurses place color-coded stickers—red, yellow, or green—on patient charts to alert physicians as to which patients are due for reassessment of telemetry status.

Cycle 4

Expanded telemetry alert/notification system.

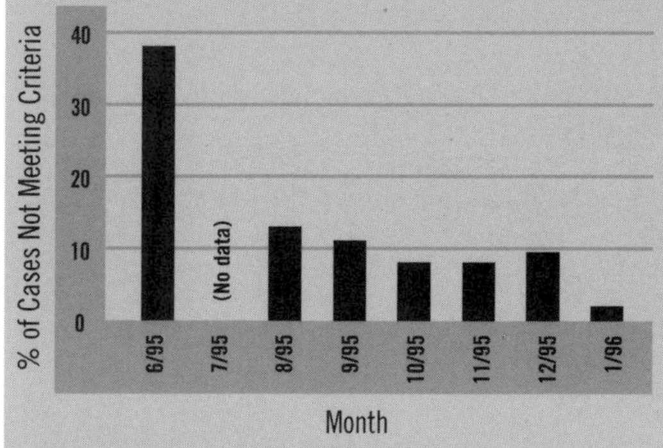

Figure 1.2
ICU/Transitional Unit Admission/Discharge Criteria

York Health System
York, PA

To learn whether the changes (cycles 1 to 4) were leading to improvement (i.e., to improved utilization of intensive care beds), the team monitored the percentage of ICU/Transitional Unit admissions that did not meet the criteria for admission and discharge. Before testing the changes, 35% of the patients on the ICU did not meet the criteria for being admitted to the ICU; after testing and implementing the changes, that number fell to below 10%.

RAMP 2: CREATE A "PULL" PROCESS FROM THE RECEIVING UNIT TO THE ED

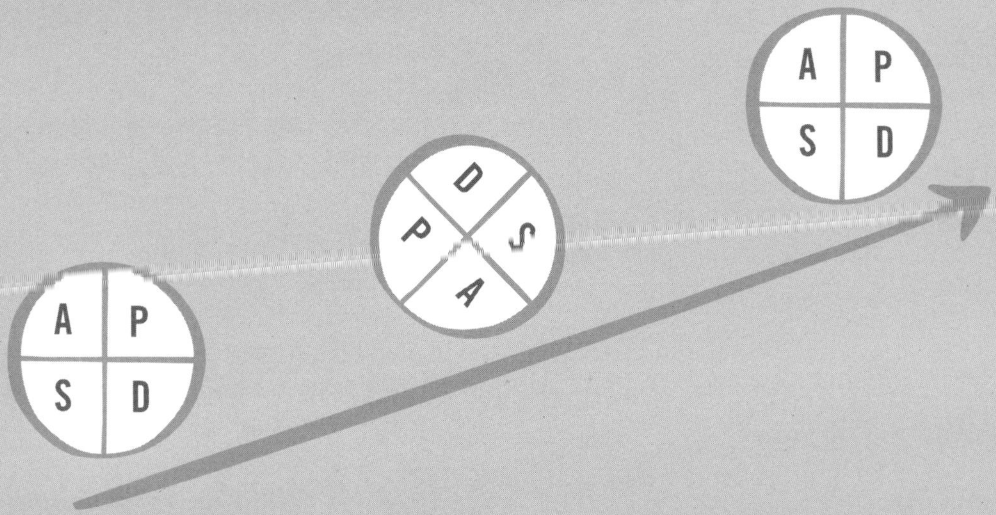

The team began working on a second hunch: streamlining the admission process and improving communication between the ED and the surgical floors would reduce patient waiting times.

Cycle 1

Tested early notification of admit.

The Emergency Department nurse pages the charge nurse on the admitting floor as soon as possible, in some cases even before the physician's decision to admit. The nurses discuss the clinical needs of the patient and the charge nurse arranges bed placement. (Note: Although this change streamlines the process, it still leaves intact the "push" system whereby the inpatient unit responds to the demand for a bed triggered by the page from the ED.)

Cycle 2

Tested Be-a-Bed-Ahead system.

Before redesign, delays occurred between the time when the ED staff notified the nurses on the surgical floor that a patient needed a bed and the time the patient was actually transferred. Under the Be-a-Bed-Ahead system, the inpatient unit anticipates the demand (by measuring demand over time) and has a bed ready into which a patient can be moved ("pulled" from the unit rather than "pushed" from the ED) as soon as the demand occurs.

Cycle 3

Expanded Be-a-Bed-Ahead system.

The outcome measure showed significant reduction in delays in transferring patients from the ED to the surgical floors.

BREAKTHROUGH IMPROVEMENT

RESULTS

York Health System reduced the time it took to transfer Emergency Department patients to inpatient beds from 66 minutes to less than 30 minutes—more than a 50% decrease.

THUS FAR IN THE GUIDE, YOU HAVE LEARNED:

Part 1

The Model for Improvement that can be applied to any area you want to improve.

Part 2

A Step-by-Step Guide to Reducing Delays and Waiting Times

In this section, you'll learn how to begin working on reducing delays and waiting times in your organization. Each step is illustrated with examples showing how organizations have used the Model for Improvement to bring about significant reductions in delays and waiting times in a short period of time.

Step One Setting Aims

Improvement begins with setting aims. An aim that is stated clearly and agreed upon by all is essential to keeping a team on track throughout its improvement efforts.

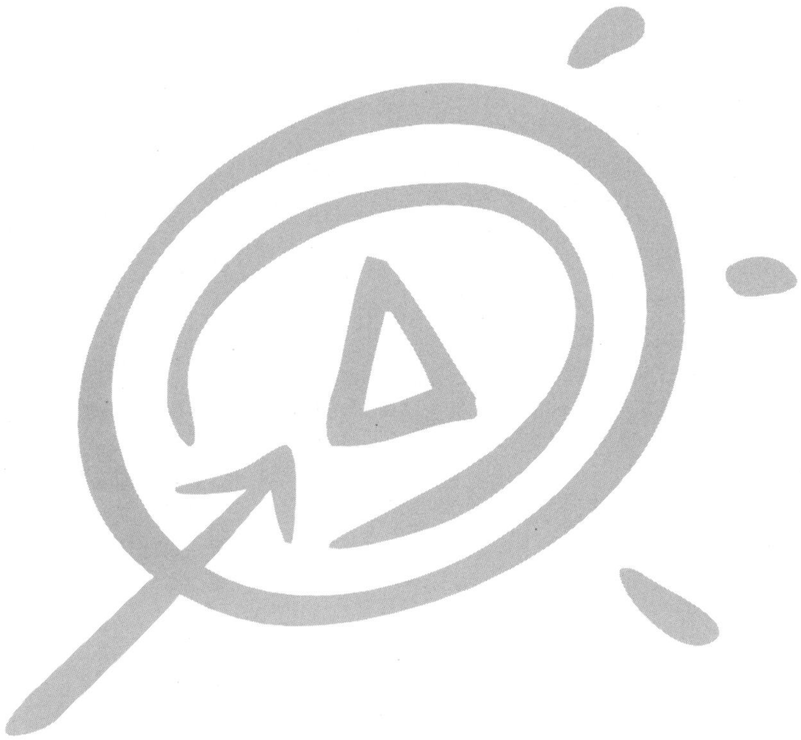

PRINCIPLES OF AN EFFECTIVE AIM STATEMENT

1. State the aim clearly.

Achieving agreement on the aim of a project is critical for maintaining progress. Teams make better progress when they are very specific about their aims.

2. Include numerical goals.

Including numerical goals can be an effective way to communicate expectations. Are small, incremental improvements expected, or are large, breakthrough changes necessary? Setting the aim "Reduce delays in surgery" is not as effective at communicating expectations as "Reduce delays in the surgery process by 50%." Including a numerical goal not only clarifies the aim; it also suggests the level of support that will be needed, and helps team members begin to think about what their measures of improvement will be and what initial changes they might make.

3. Set stretch goals.

Setting stretch goals—for example, "Reduce delays in the surgery process by 50%"—clarifies immediately that maintaining the status quo is not an option. One role of leadership is to serve notice that the goal cannot be met by tweaking the existing system. Once this is clear, people begin to look for ways to overcome barriers to achieving the stretch goals.

4. Avoid aim drift.

Once the aim has been set, the team needs to be careful not to back away from it. What was initially a stretch goal—"Reduce delays in the surgery process by 50%"—can slip almost imperceptibly to "Reduce delays in the surgery process by 40%," or "by 20%." One way to avoid this is to repeat the aim continually; start each team meeting with an explicit statement of aim, for example, "Remember, we're here to reduce delays in the surgery process by 50%."

5. Be prepared to refocus aim.

Every team needs to recognize when to refocus its aim. If the team's overall aim is at a system level (e.g., "Reduce waiting times for all patients coming to Ambulatory Care Services for outpatient testing by 50%"), the team's members may find that focusing for a time on a specific subsystem (e.g., "Reduce waiting times for cardiology patients coming to Ambulatory Care Services for outpatient testing by 50%") will help them achieve the desired system-level goal. Note: Don't confuse "aim drift" (backing away from the initial aim) with consciously deciding to refocus the initial aim.

1 Sewickley Valley Hospital, Sewickley, PA

Reducing Delays in Surgery

Background: Sewickley Valley Hospital is a 225-bed community hospital located in Sewickley, PA. It has six operating rooms and performs approximately 6,500 surgeries per year. At the beginning of the project, scheduled start times in the operating rooms were delayed 95% to 100% of the time.

2 Chester County Hospital, West Chester, PA

Reducing Delays in the Emergency Department

Background: Before May 1995, Chester County Hospital in West Chester, PA, had experienced an increase in the number of patients leaving the Emergency Department without being treated. This was due to long waiting times before patients were seen by a physician, as well as long delays in patients being transferred from the ED to inpatient beds.

EXAMPLES OF EFFECTIVE AIM STATEMENTS

Aim (1): Reduce delays in surgical services for patients on the day of surgery. Assure that the actual incision is made within 90 minutes after arrival for all outpatients.

Aim (2): Reduce patients' actual and perceived waiting time in the Emergency Department. Develop a separate process for treating patients with nonemergent, uncomplicated illnesses and injuries that would reduce that subpopulation's waiting time by 50%.

AIM

3 Deborah Heart and Lung Center Browns Mills, NJ

Reducing Waiting Times in Clinics and Physicians' Offices

Background: Deborah Heart and Lung Center (DHLC) is a cardiovascular and pulmonary specialty hospital in southern New Jersey. The Ambulatory Care Services (ACS) treats 25,000 outpatients annually in nine clinics, up from 14,000 outpatients in 1992. Outpatients found waiting times too long.

Aim: Reduce the waiting time for patients coming to Ambulatory Care Services for outpatient testing by 50%. At the beginning of the project, patients spent an average of 198 minutes at the Ambulatory Care Services for a first evaluation. Of that time, 93 minutes were spent in actual evaluation and 105 minutes were spent waiting.

4 MetroHealth Indianapolis, IN

Increasing Access to Care

Background: MetroHealth is a multi-specialty group, part of the Methodist Medical Group in central Indiana, delivering mostly primary care. A customer satisfaction survey conducted in 1994 indicated that access to routine primary care appointments needed improvement. Patients were asked to rate the length of time they had to wait for an appointment; 38% of those waiting longer than one week rated this wait as "poor to fair."

Aim: Improve access to routine primary care appointments. Develop a process by which 90% of members requesting a nonurgent primary care appointment are offered an appointment with a physician within one week of their request.

Step Two Forming the Team

Getting the right people on the team is critical to a successful improvement effort. Teams vary in size and composition; each organization builds teams to suit its own needs.

It is important for the team to include a mixture of representatives such as physicians, nurses, managers, and administrators.

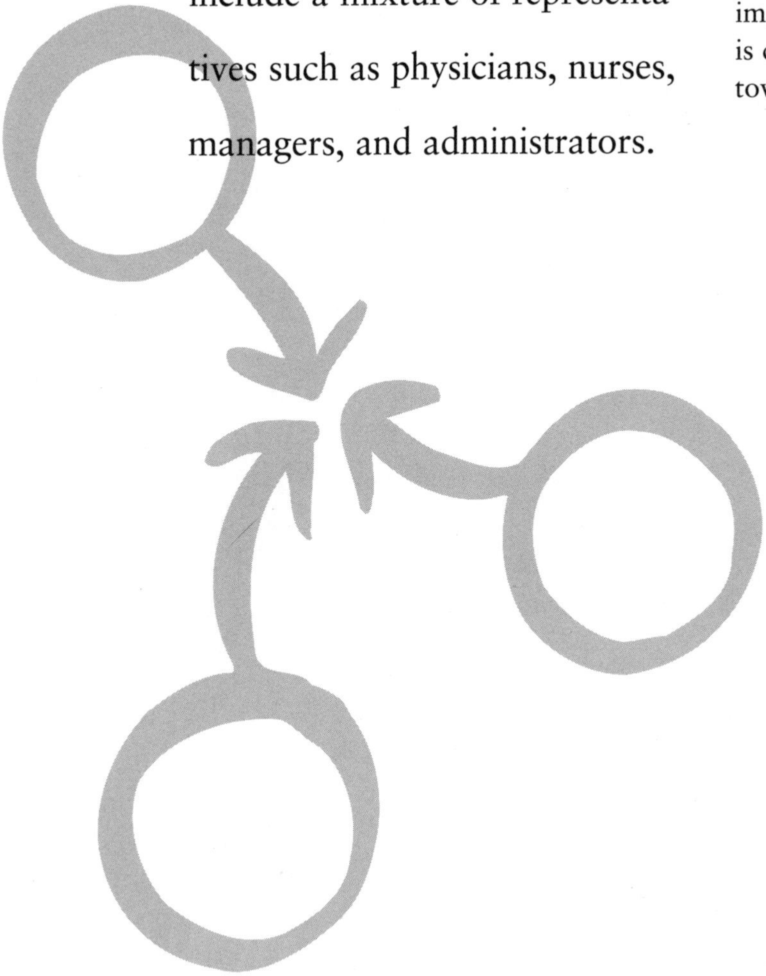

A team's composition depends upon its aim:

First, review the aim.

Second, consider the system that relates to that aim: what processes will be affected by the improvement?

Third, be sure that the team includes the appropriate individuals to drive improvement in those areas.

The team should be able to meet relatively frequently, to work efficiently, and to institute change in the organization quickly. Perhaps the single most important success factor of a team is commitment to working together toward a shared goal.

THREE INGREDIENTS OF AN EFFECTIVE TEAM

Effective teams should have representation from three different areas of expertise within the organization. There may be one or more individuals on the team who represent each of the areas, or one individual may represent more than one area, but all three areas should be represented in order to drive change successfully in the organization.

System Leadership

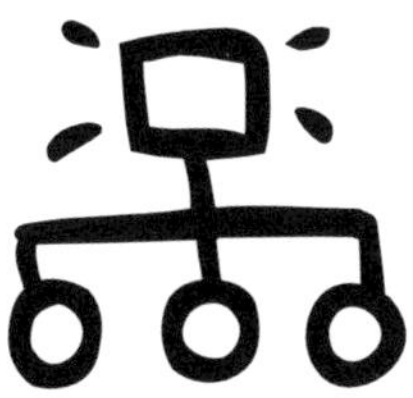

Teams need someone with enough clout in the organization to institute a change; when a change is suggested, this person has the authority to get it done. It is important that this person have authority in all of the areas that are affected by the change. In addition, this individual should have the authority to allocate the time and resources necessary to the team to achieve its aim.

Technical Expertise

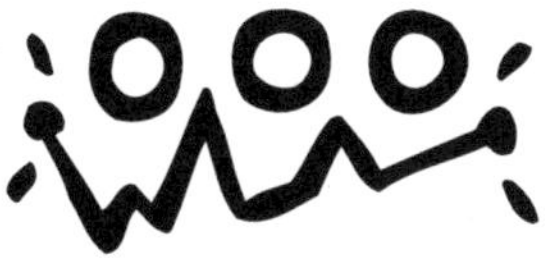

Teams need a subject matter expert, someone who understands the entire process of care that is being improved. Additional technical support may be provided by an expert on improvement methods who can help the team understand what to measure, how to design tests of change, how to collect and display data, and how to understand the information contained in the data.

Day-to-Day Leadership

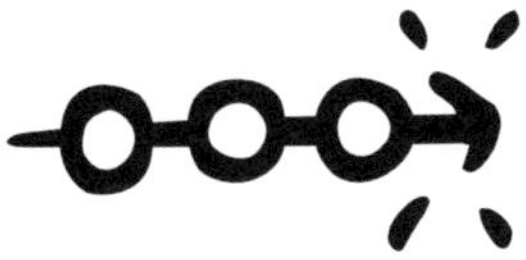

Teams also need someone who works on a daily basis in the process that is being improved and thus understands the process thoroughly. This person should also understand the various effects of planned changes in the process and have the desire and ability to drive the project on a daily basis.

EXAMPLES OF EFFECTIVE TEAMS

1 Sewickley Valley Hospital
Sewickley, PA

Aim: Reduce delays in surgical services for patients on the day of surgery: incision within 90 minutes of arrival for all outpatients.

Team:

- Nurse Manager, Operating Room
- Nurse Manager, Outpatient Surgery
- Anesthesiologist
- Perioperative Facilitator
- Nurse, Operating Room
- Nurse, Post Anesthesia Care Unit
- Certified Registered Nurse Anesthetist (CRNA)

In support of the team:

Surgeon

Hospital Administrator

2 Chester County Hospital
West Chester, PA

Aim: Reduce patients' actual and perceived waiting time in the Emergency Department. Reduce the waiting time for nonemergent patients by 50%.

Team:

- Nurse Manager, ED
- Medical Director, ED
- Nurses from all three shifts
- Patient Care Assistant
- Unit Secretary
- Paramedic Manager
- Process Improvement Coordinator

In support of the team:

Chief Operating Officer

Nurse Executive

TEAM

3 Deborah Heart and Lung Center Browns Mills, NJ

Aim: Reduce the waiting time for patients coming to Ambulatory Care Services (ACS) for outpatient testing by 50%.

Team:

- Physician (Chair, Department of Cardiology)
- Physician (Chair, QA/UR Committee)
- Assistant Director, Nursing for Clinical Practice
- ACS scheduling clerk

Matching Team and Aim:
Deborah Heart and Lung Center

After testing some initial changes, the team realized that it would be more successful if it concentrated on making changes within the cardiology area of Ambulatory Care Services, rather than trying to change the entire system. The chief of cardiology, a member of the team, could then function as the system leader since he had authority over cardiology but not over all of ambulatory care. The project was now more manageable, and the team membership had the authority to make the necessary changes.

4 MetroHealth Indianapolis, IN

Aim: Improve access to routine primary care appointments: offer non-urgent appointments within one week of the request 90% of the time.

Team:

- CQI Coordinator
- Clinical Administrator, RN
- Reception Coordinator
- Physician, Adult Internal Medicine
- Physician Assistant
- Health Center Administrator

In support of the team:

Medical Director

Site Lead Physician

Pediatrician (expert on data collection)

Step Three Establishing Measures

Once the aim has been set and the team has been formed, the next step is to establish measures that will indicate if a change leads to an improvement. If a team has done a good job of articulating its aim, it is not difficult to plan simple, effective measures.

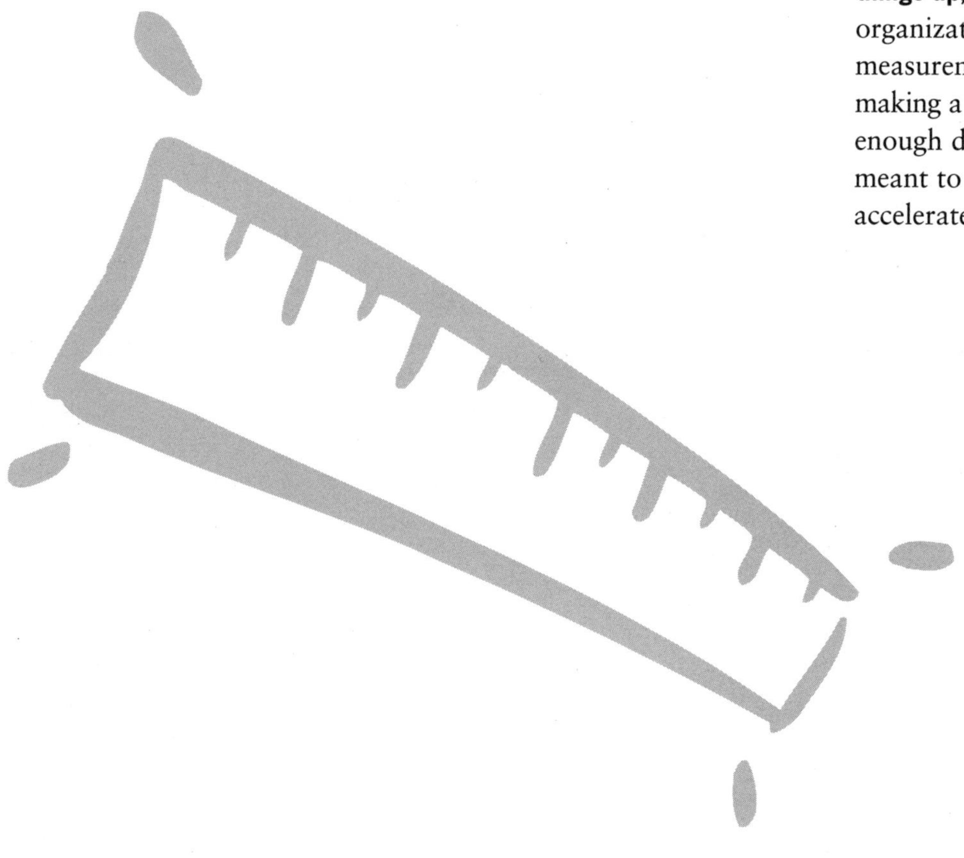

Teams usually need to track both outcome and process measures:

Outcome measures tell a team whether the changes it is making are actually leading to improvement—that is, helping to achieve the stated aim.

Process measures tell a team whether a specific process change has been accomplished and whether it is having the intended effect. A team often establishes several process measures in the course of its work. The assumption is that improvement in a process measure will have an eventual impact on the outcome measure.

Measurement should be used to speed things up, not to slow them down. Many organizations get bogged down in measurement, delaying the move to making a change until they have collected enough data. The following tips are meant to help teams use measures to accelerate improvement.

TIPS FOR EFFECTIVE MEASUREMENT

1. Seek usefulness, not perfection.

Remember, measurement is not the goal; improvement is the goal. A team needs just enough measurement to know whether changes are leading to improvement, in order to move forward to the next step.

2. Don't wait for the information system.

Lots of useful information already exists, or is relatively simple to get. Don't wait for the financial figures to come out two months from now, or for the surveys to come back in two weeks.

3. Use sampling.

Sampling is a simple, powerful way to help understand how a system is working. Instead of measuring all of something, measure a sample—every 10th patient, or the next 10 patients, or the next 30 bills.

4. Use qualitative and quantitative data.

For example, rather than delaying testing a change until the data collection about delays in the ICU is complete, ask the ICU nurses, "What are the top three or four reasons for delays in admitting?" These qualitative judgments can be verified and data can be collected during tests of change.

5. Use a balanced set of measures.

Use balancing measures to make sure that changes being made to improve one part of the system aren't causing new problems in other parts of the system. For example, reducing length of stay may cause an increase in readmissions; increasing access to same-day appointments may cause longer waiting times in the physician's office.

6. Use outcome and process measures.

For example, if the aim is reducing waiting times in the ED, an outcome measure might be the duration of the ED visit. Process measures might be the accuracy of registration information or the availability of x-rays at the time of the physician's exam.

7. Plot data over time.

Improvement requires change, and change is by definition a temporal phenomenon. Much of the information about a system and how to improve it can be obtained by plotting data—on cost, health outcomes, delays, and patient satisfaction—over time and observing trends and other patterns.

1 Sewickley Valley Hospital Sewickley, PA

Aim: Reduce delays in surgical services for patients on the day of surgery: incision within 90 minutes of arrival for all outpatients.

2 Chester County Hospital West Chester, PA

Aim: Reduce patients' actual and perceived waiting time in the Emergency Department. Reduce the waiting time for nonemergent patients by 50%.

EXAMPLES OF EFFECTIVE MEASURES

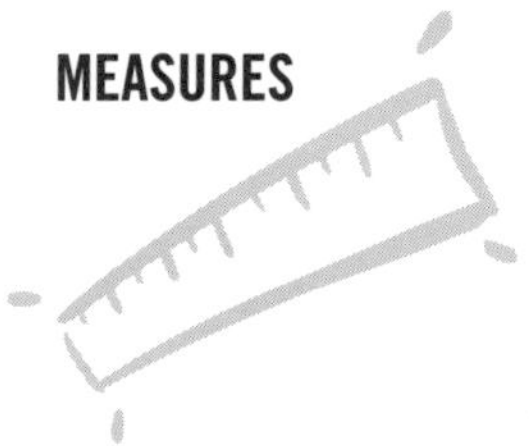

Outcome Measure:

Figure 2.1

MEDIAN DELAY IN SURGERY: 11 AM AND 2 PM

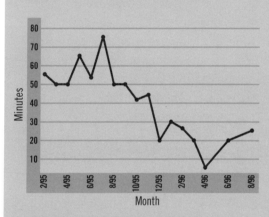

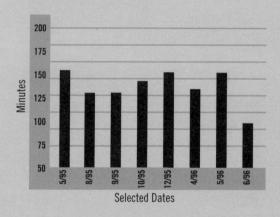

The team measured the difference between scheduled start time for surgery and actual start time. Instead of measuring delays in all surgical cases, the team used sampling to simplify measurement: they measured delays at 11 AM and 2 PM in each operating room, one day per week, and then used the data to plot median delay. The 11 AM point is most likely to reflect delays that occur in the morning cases, and the 2 PM point reflects delays that occur in the afternoon cases.

Outcome Measure:

Figure 2.2

ED AVERAGE DISCHARGE TIME

The team measured "average discharge time," starting with the time the patient enters the ED and ending with the time the patient is either admitted to an inpatient unit or discharged from the facility.

MEASURES

3 Deborah Heart and Lung Center Browns Mills, NJ

Aim: Reduce the waiting time for patients coming to Ambulatory Care Services (ACS) for outpatient testing by 50%.

Outcome Measure:

Figure 2.3

WAITING TIME IN CARDIOLOGY CLINIC

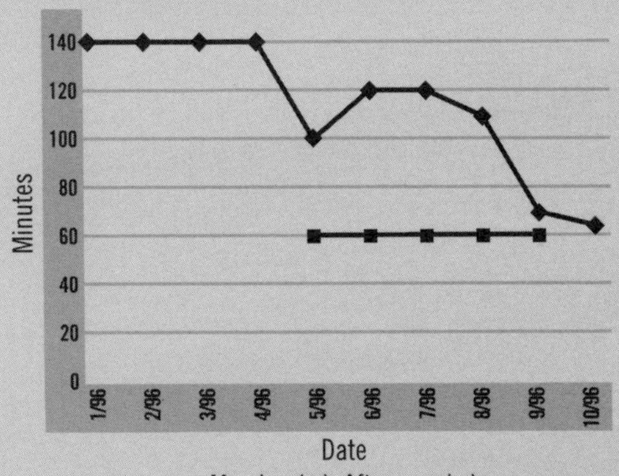

Morning (◆), Afternoon (■)

The team measured the amount of time patients spent waiting in the cardiology clinic. They computed waiting time by subtracting an estimate of the process time from the overall length of the visit. Note that the addition of afternoon clinics, beginning in May 1996, caused a decrease in waiting times in the morning by shifting patients to the afternoon.

4 MetroHealth Indianapolis, IN

Aim: Improve access to routine primary care appointments: offer non-urgent appointments within one week of the request 90% of the time.

Outcome Measure:

Figure 2.4

ACCESS TO ROUTINE PEDIATRIC APPOINTMENTS

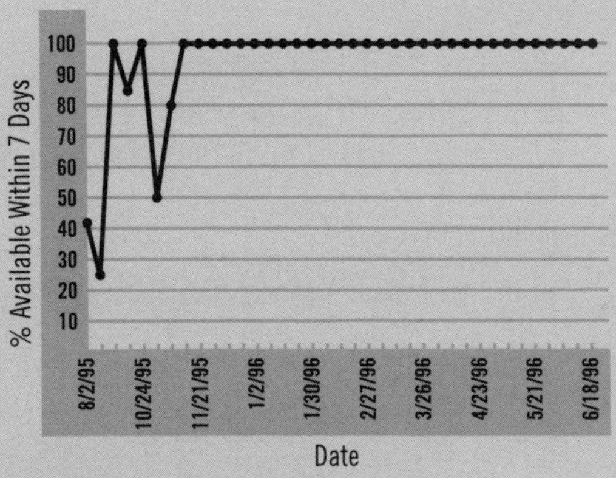

The team collected baseline data at a test site on routine pediatric appointment availability. Before the team made changes, only 42% of patients were offered a routine appointment with a physician within seven days.

Step Four Developing and Testing

DEVELOPING CHANGES: REDUCING DELAYS IN SURGERY

1 Sewickley Valley Hospital
Sewickley, PA

Once you have set a clear aim, formed the right team, and established simple measures to indicate if a change leads to an improvement, the next step is to develop and test changes. Sewickley Valley Hospital exemplifies developing and testing several different ideas for change simultaneously. Chester County Hospital shows how one cycle can be linked to another to test and refine a change.

Aim: Reduce delays in surgical services for patients on the day of surgery: incision within 90 minutes of arrival for all outpatients.

Sewickley Valley Hospital's team developed a series of changes and tested them in three surgical subprocesses—Outpatient Surgery (OPS), Preoperative Holding, and Operating Room (OR). The team used many of the "change concepts" described in Part 3 of this Guide to come up with ideas for promising changes.

Key change concept used throughout the project: 4 Synchronize

Process change: The team defined incision time as the key reference point in the process and timed all of the subtasks in the surgery process relative to the incision time. In order to achieve synchronization, the team applied several other change concepts.

A. Outpatient Surgery

Change concept: 3 Minimize Handoffs

Process change: Previously, nurses' aides from the OR transported patients from Outpatient Surgery, where registration for surgery patients takes place, to Preoperative Holding. Now staff in Outpatient Surgery transport patients both to Preoperative Holding and directly to the OR when needed, freeing OR nurses' aides for other tasks in the OR.

Change concept: 8 Consider People to Be in the Same System

Process change: Previously, a bottleneck would occur if the anesthesiologist assigned to OPS was backed up with patient assessments. Now the anesthesiologists in the OR are beeped to assist the OPS anesthesiologist in preoperative assessments.

Changes

Change concept: 24 Identify and Manage the Constraint

Change concept: 1 Do Tasks in Parallel

Process change: Previously, the anesthesiologist waited for the nurse to complete the nursing assessment before beginning the anesthesiology assessment. Now, if free, the anesthesiologist performs an assessment before the nurse does; in some cases, they may perform their assessments at the same time.

Note: For a comprehensive list of ideas for change, including a more detailed description of the change concepts used here, see Part 3, 27 Change Concepts for Reducing Delays and Waiting Times.

B. Preoperative Holding

Change concept: 7 Use Automation

Process change: The preoperative facilitator coordinates the movement of patients from Outpatient Surgery, to Preoperative Holding, to the OR. To enhance communication, the facilitator now carries a portable phone to be notified when a prior case is finishing or when a patient is being moved from OPS to Preoperative Holding. In addition, OR nurses' aides carry beepers to let them know when patients are ready to be moved from one area to another or when they are needed for other duties.

C. Operating Room

Change concept: 1 Do Tasks in Parallel

Process change: Previously, OR nurses, Certified Registered Nurse Anesthetists (CRNAs), and anesthesiologists worked with the patient sequentially. Now they work with the patient simultaneously, completing anesthesia assessments and preparing the patient for surgery. For example, the CRNA assists with starting the IV while the nurse completes the assessment. Room set-up, which had been done prior to preparing the patient for surgery, is now also done simultaneously with preparing the patient.

Change concept: 21 Improve Predictions

Process change: Previously, delays occurred when cases were scheduled too close together because scheduling was based on how long a procedure was supposed to take rather than on how long it actually took. Now cases are scheduled with realistic start times based on measures of actual case lengths.

TESTING CHANGES: REDUCING DELAYS IN THE EMERGENCY DEPARTMENT

2 Chester County Hospital West Chester, PA

Aim: Reduce patients' actual and perceived waiting time in the Emergency Department. Reduce the waiting time for nonemergent patients by 50%.

Chester County Hospital's team used the change concept, "Use Multiple Processes," to institute a "Med Express" system that identifies patients with nonemergent, uncomplicated illnesses and injuries (e.g., suture removals, minor cuts, etc.) at the point of triage. Previously, every patient coming into the Emergency Department went through the same process. Ramp 1 shows how the team tested the Med Express system for patients requiring less complicated treatment, thereby reducing delays not only for them, but for all ED patients.

In addition, the team discovered that significant delays occurred when patients were transferred from the Emergency Department to inpatient units. In order to reduce delays in the ED, staff of both the ED and the inpatient units needed to recognize that they were part of the same system (change concept, "Consider People to Be in the Same System") and work together. Ramp 2 shows how the team used the change concept, "Use Pull Systems," to reduce delays when transferring patients from the ED to inpatient units.

Measure

Figure 2.5
MED EXPRESS CYCLE TIME

Chester County Hospital
West Chester, PA

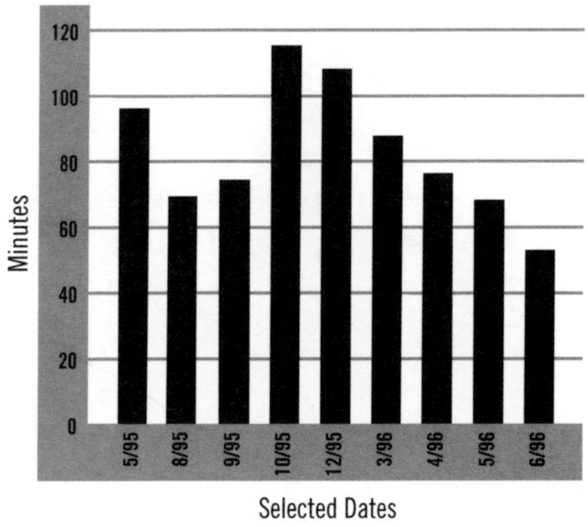

While testing the Med Express system, the team measured Med Express Cycle Time: the interval between the time of a patient's admission to the Emergency Department and the time of discharge home.

Ramp 1: Develop a system to identify patients with nonemergent, uncomplicated injuries at the point of triage.

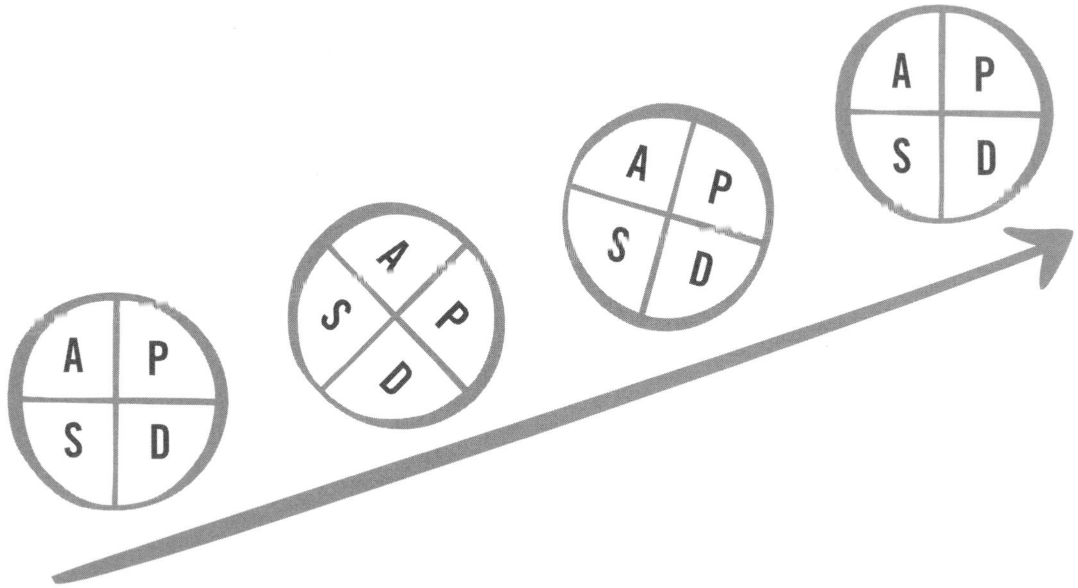

Cycle 1

Develop and test Med Express system.

Identify nonemergent patients at point of triage, mark paperwork with a green dot and place it on a green fluorescent clipboard. Coding system allows healthcare team to identify patients easily. A physician sees Med Express patients out of order of arrival and whenever time permits, especially while waiting for test results on emergent patients.

Cycle 2

Develop and test guidelines for Med Express.

Develop written guidelines for Med Express patients. Educate entire healthcare team on written guidelines. Notify ancillary departments (lab and radiology) about Med Express efforts. Incorporate guidelines into system.

Cycle 3

Improve radiology response time.

Look at lab turnaround times and radiology turnaround times. Radiology looks for ways to increase response time. Radiology techs begin to wear beepers on all three shifts to be alerted to need of ED x-ray and to be paged as a resource in ordering correct radiology film.

Cycle 4

Increase triage coverage during peak hours.

Team measures waiting times at different times of day, and discovers especially long delays during evening hours. Triage currently runs from 10 AM to 10 PM. Provide additional triage coverage during peak evening hours.

Ramp 2: Develop a system to "pull" patients from the Emergency Department to the receiving unit.

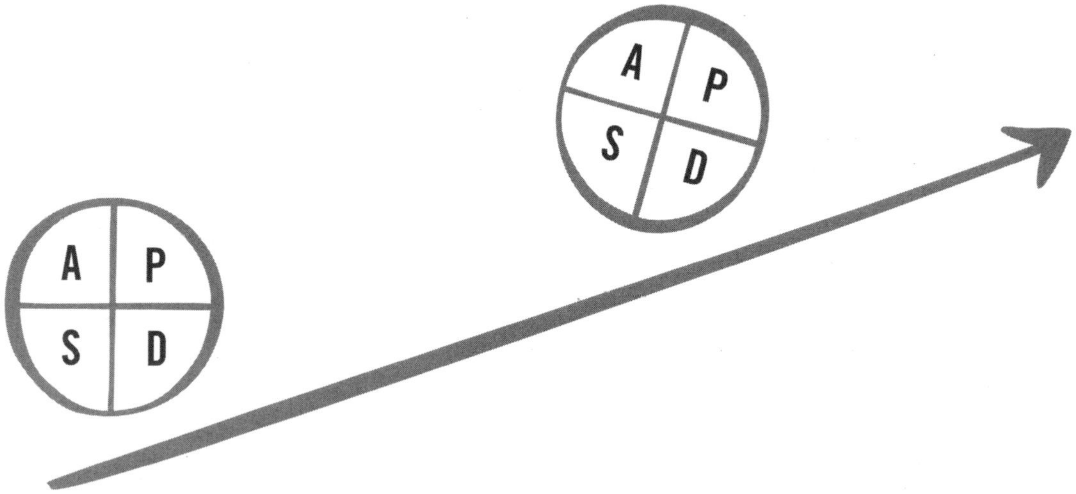

Cycle 1

Delays in the ED are related to delays in receiving units.

In the course of cycles run as part of Ramp 1, the team discovers that delays are occurring in the ED because inpatient units do not have beds open. When a patient needs to be admitted to the hospital, the ED notifies the receiving unit and waits until a bed is available.

Cycle 2

Develop and test a Be-a-Bed-Ahead system.

In a Be-a-Bed-Ahead system, admissions identifies the next female and male beds ready to be filled, and notifies the nursing staff and housekeeping staff. In this way, ED patients are "pulled to" the unit instead of being "pushed from" the ED.

Results: Breakthrough Improvement Within 12 Months

By moving Emergency Department patients into multiple processes, Chester County Hospital has reduced cycle time for Med Express patients from 98 minutes to 39 minutes—a reduction of 59%.

In addition, waiting time for all patients in the ED to see a physician has been reduced from an average of 66 minutes to an average of 39 minutes—a reduction of approximately 30%. ED patients who need to be admitted now wait an average of 61 minutes from the decision to admit until actual transfer to an inpatient unit, versus an average of 81 minutes in May 1995—a reduction of approximately 20%.

TIPS FOR SUCCESSFUL TESTS OF CHANGE

1. Stay a cycle ahead. When designing a test, imagine at the start what the subsequent test or two might be, given various possible findings in the "Study" phase.

2. Vary design parameters to accelerate testing. Common variables that can be scaled down to permit testing include the following: number of patients, doctors, and others involved in the test (e.g., "Sample the next 10" instead of "Get a sample of 200"); number of units, beds, locations involved in the test (e.g., "Try it on 6 West" instead of "Try it on the medical service").

3. Pick willing volunteers (e.g., "I know Dr. Jones will help us" instead of "How can we convince Dr. Smith to buy in?").

4. Avoid the need for consensus, buy-in, or political solution during the early testing phase. Save these for later stages.

5. Don't reinvent the wheel. Instead, replicate changes made elsewhere (e.g., use someone else's questionnaire without revising it).

6. Pick easy changes to try. Look for the concepts that seem most feasible.

7. Avoid technical slowdowns (e.g., don't wait for the new computer to arrive; try paper and pencil instead).

8. Stay aware of the underlying concept being tested. If possible, work "forward" from the concept, not "backward" from the change. (For example, in working on improving access to primary care, it may be better to ask, "What process changes could ease the bottleneck of physicians?" than to start with the idea, "Let's hire more physicians to cover peak times.")

9. Be prepared to close down a ramp. One reason to test is to discover whether a particular series of process changes fulfills its goal. If tests are not yielding results, they should be stopped. This is not "failure," but rather "learning." It happens to most successful teams.

THUS FAR IN THE GUIDE, YOU HAVE LEARNED:

Part 1 *The Model for Improvement that can be applied to any area you want to improve.*

Part 2 *A step-by-step guide to using that model to work on reducing delays and waiting times, with each of the basic steps—setting aims, forming the team, establishing measures, and developing and testing changes—illustrated with examples.*

Part 3

27 Change Concepts for Reducing Delays and Waiting Times

In this section, you will learn three basic strategies for reducing delays and waiting times and, for each of those strategies, a group of change concepts that you can use to generate good ideas for changes.

Three Strategies for Reducing Delays

In order to make changes to reduce delays and waiting times, it is important to understand the basic dynamics that cause delays in any system. Delays occur at a variety of different times, including the following: when processes that happen simultaneously are not synchronized; when sequential steps have ineffective hand-offs; and when the demand on a system exceeds the capacity of that system.

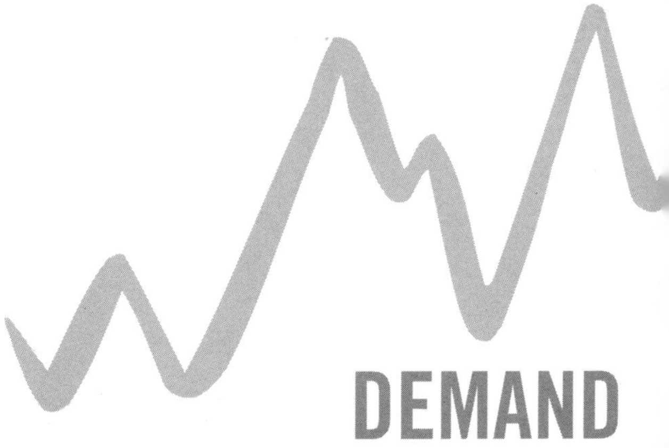

TO REDUCE DELAYS AND WAITING TIMES, USE

1. Redesign the system.

There are several ways to make a system more efficient, thereby increasing its capacity without adding resources. System redesign involves changing one or more of the processes, or sets of tasks, that make up the system. Relatively simple changes can make a system more efficient and less prone to delays: tasks that traditionally have been done in sequence can be done concurrently, handoffs can be eliminated, tasks can be synchronized around a common reference point, steps can be removed or rearranged.

- For example, an emergency department redesigns its system for ordering x-rays as follows: instead of having patients go through triage, registration, rooming, nurse assessment, and physician evaluation before any ordering of x-rays, the emergency department now has patients see a triage nurse upon arrival. The triage nurse orders x-rays as needed, x-rays are performed, and results are available at the time of physician evaluation.

and Waiting Times

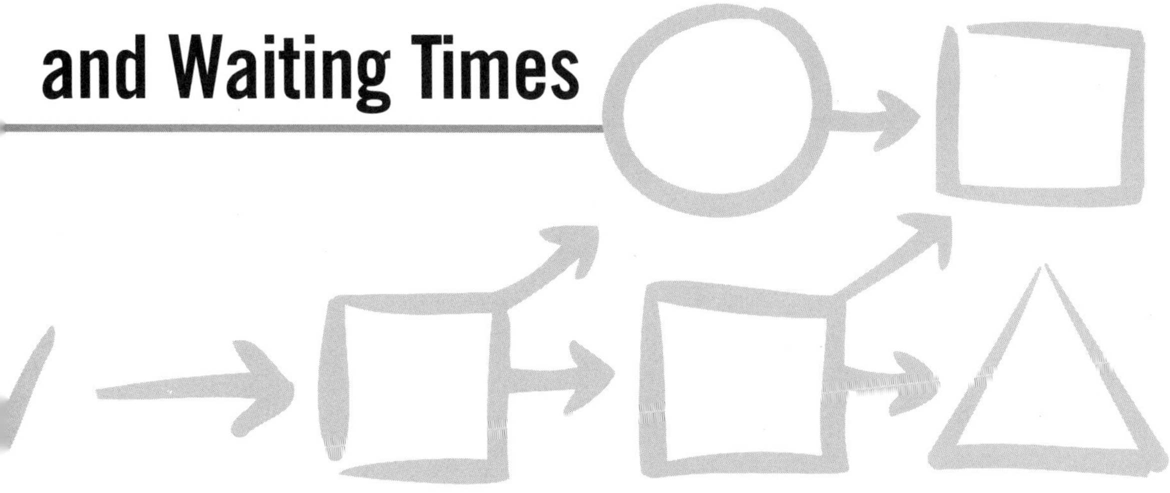

SYSTEM

ONE OR MORE OF THE FOLLOWING STRATEGIES:

2. Shape the demand.

Instead of adding capacity to a system, delays can often be reduced by shaping demand. This can be accomplished by a variety of methods:

- Extinguishing the demand for ineffective care. For example, instead of automatically scheduling recheck appointments following an office visit for an acute problem, give the patient a reminder to phone after a predetermined time interval to reevaluate the need for the recheck appointment.
- Substituting a service by providing the service in another location or in another way. For example, instead of scheduling individual appointments, offer group appointments for patients with hypertension.
- Reframing the need so that the customer of the service no longer perceives a need for the service. For example, reduce the frequency of required camp physicals from every year to once every two years.

3. Match capacity to demand.

Not only does demand for care vary, but often capacity varies from hour to hour and week to week. Sometimes fairly simple changes can be made to bring the capacity of the system into alignment with demand. Such measures do not necessarily require major redesign of the system but may involve simpler steps such as readjusting the current capacity to match the peak demand times. Some examples:

- A clinic with long waiting room waits does not hire additional physicians; rather, the clinic assigns more of its physicians to those times when patient demand for urgent care is highest.
- A nursing unit with delays because admissions from the ED coincide with the time when patients are being discharged from the unit redesigns the process so that discharge takes place before the busy admission time.

Understanding System Capacity

HOW TO DETERMINE DEMAND

The demand on a system can be measured simply—by hour of the day, day of the week, month of the year. Basic sampling is all that's needed. Figure 3.1 shows the average number of patients seen in an emergency department per hour, for each hour of the day. It shows that demand is relatively low during the first seven hours, and relatively high during hours 18 to 21.

Figure 3.1
EMERGENCY DEPARTMENT DEMAND BY HOUR

Sample Figure

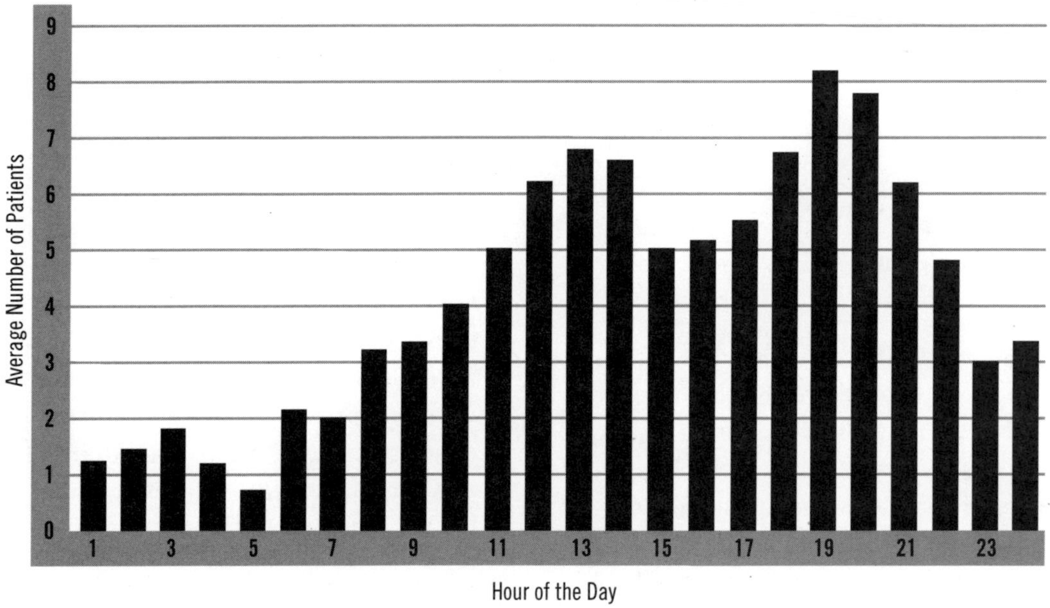

and Demand

HOW TO DETERMINE CAPACITY

The capacity of a system can be measured similarly. Figure 3.2 shows the number of physicians available at a clinic per each half day over a period of two weeks. The clinic was surprised to discover the amount of variation in its capacity.

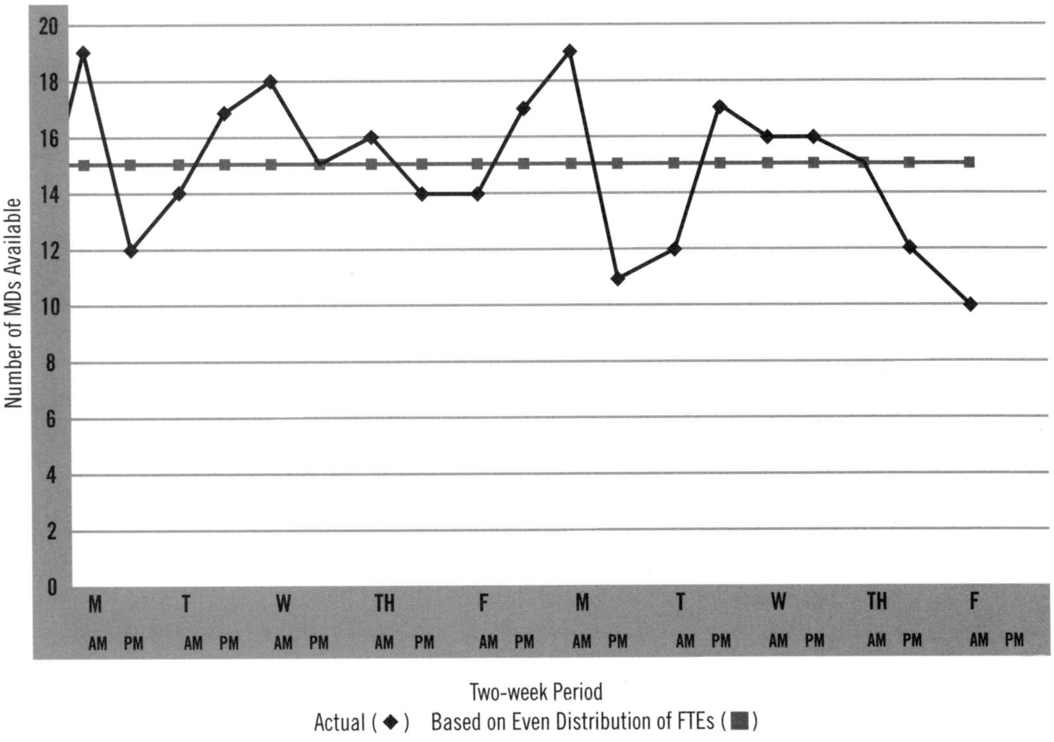

Figure 3.2
PROVIDERS AVAILABLE

Virginia Mason
Medical Center
Seattle, WA

HOW TO IDENTIFY THE CONSTRAINT

Not every process in a system has the same capacity. A constraint (also called a bottleneck) is that part of the system that has the smallest capacity relative to the demand on it. If changes are made to improve parts of a system without addressing the constraint, the changes may not result in reduction of delays and waiting times for the entire system.

To identify the constraint, observe where the work is piling up or where the lines are forming. Alternatively, do some simple calculations; for example, Figure 3.3 shows the capacity of the five processes in a preoperative clinic. Note that the chart identifies the nurse as the constraint.

HOW TO MANAGE THE CONSTRAINT

Constraints should not have idle time.	**Dx:** The physician is in the exam room waiting to see the first patient of the day while the patient is being registered.
If experts are the constraint, they should only be doing work for which an expert is needed.	**Dx:** In preoperative testing, patients are backed up waiting for the nurse (the constraint in the process).
To increase the capacity of the constraint, give some of the work to nonconstraints, even if it is less "efficient" for the nonconstraints.	**Dx:** The ophthalmologist writes up notes after the patient visit.
Put inspection in front of a constraint.	**Dx:** On the day of surgery, key x-rays are not available.

	Anesthesia	Nursing	Phlebotomy	EKG	X-ray
Total process minutes including paperwork	15 min	18 min	8 min	10 min	9 min
Estimated capacity (number of visits per day) with breaks, calls, lunch	48 visits	36 visits	58 visits	42 visits	on call
Range of visits per day (4-day period)	27–45 visits	23–38 visits	22–41 visits	11–30 visits	7–21 visits
Average number of visits per day (4-day period)	35 visits	27 visits	29 visits	20 visits	14 visits

Figure 3.3
PREOP CLINIC CAPACITY

Beth Israel Deaconess
Medical Center–East
Campus
Boston, MA

Rx: Register the patient after the exam.

Rx: The receptionist or assistant assumes tasks that are being done by the nurse, but do not require nursing skills.

Rx: The assistant takes dictation during the ophthalmology exam.

Rx: One person coordinates and expedites all necessary information on the day before surgery.

HOW TO MEASURE DELAYS

Cycle time is the elapsed time from the start of a process at a defined beginning to the completion of the process at a defined end.

Cycle time is the sum of process time and waiting time. Figure 3.4 shows the total cycle time for preprocedure testing; it indicates what part of that time was spent in the various substantive steps of the preprocedure testing process (process time) and what part of that time was spent waiting.

Figure 3.4
PREPROCEDURE TESTING: CYCLE TIME = PROCESS TIME + WAITING TIME

Beth Israel Deaconess Medical Center–East Campus
Boston, MA

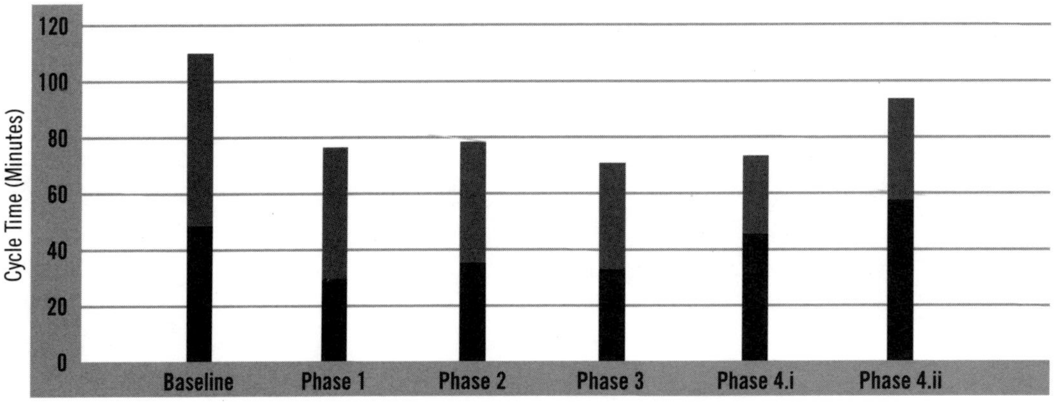

Waiting Time (■) vs. Process Time (■)

There are a variety of ways to estimate how much of the cycle time is process time and how much is waiting time. The following are some methods for doing this, listed in decreasing order of rigor:

- Conduct a time study that records the beginning and ending times of each step in the process, as well as the overall cycle time.
- Measure the overall cycle time. To estimate process time, measure the time for each step in the process by sampling a few patients or by asking workers in the process to estimate the duration of their step. To determine waiting time, subtract the estimated process time from the overall cycle time.
- Use an heuristic approach based on a "group of size 1." Estimate how long the process would take if there were only one patient, one sample, or one invoice in the system. It is assumed that the waiting time derives from the complexity introduced by large numbers of people, samples, or information flowing at the same time. Therefore, subtract the estimate of process time from the overall cycle time to estimate waiting time.

HOW TO USE A CHANGE CONCEPT TO PLAN A PROCESS CHANGE

- A change concept is a general, scientifically grounded idea for change.
- A process change is the specific, "physical" realization of that idea in a local context.
- The change which is then tested in a small-scale Plan-Do-Study-Act cycle.

Here is how one organization used a change concept to develop a process change:

Sewickley Valley Hospital, in Sewickley, PA, set the following aim:

Aim: Reduce delays on day of surgery by 50%.

In answering the question, "What change can we make that will result in an improvement," the team selected the following change concept:

Change concept: 1 Do Tasks in Parallel

The team used the change concept to develop the following process change:

Process change: Instead of setting up instruments in the operating room and then preparing the patient for surgery, perform these two tasks simultaneously.

The team then tested the process change in the following small-scale Plan-Do-Study-Act cycle:

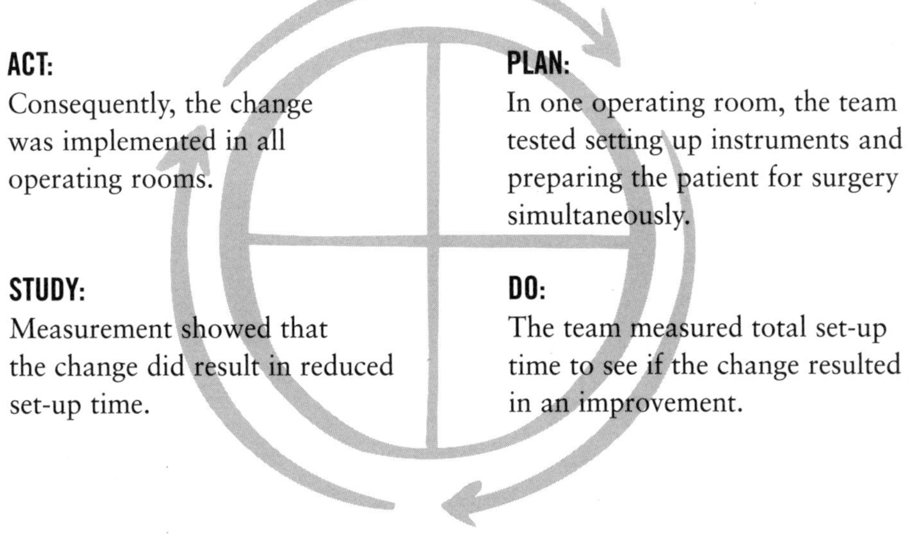

ACT:
Consequently, the change was implemented in all operating rooms.
PLAN:
In one operating room, the team tested setting up instruments and preparing the patient for surgery simultaneously.
STUDY:
Measurement showed that the change did result in reduced set-up time.
DO:
The team measured total set-up time to see if the change resulted in an improvement.

27 Change Concepts for Reducing

You can use the following list of change concepts to develop good ideas for process changes that will lead to rapid, significant improvements. Each change concept is followed by examples of specific process changes based on the concept.

The list is organized according to the three core strategies for reducing delays and waiting times: redesign the system, shape the demand, and match capacity to demand.

See Part 4 for examples of the application of these change concepts to reducing delays and waiting times in surgery, the emergency department, and clinics and physicians' offices, and to increasing access to care.

Note: The change concepts were initially developed by Tom Nolan and colleagues at Associates in Process Improvement as a resource for developing ideas for changes in a variety of business contexts (see Langley G, Nolan K, Nolan T, Norman C, Provost L. *The Improvement Guide: A Practical Approach to Enhancing Organizational Performance.* San Francisco: Jossey-Bass Publishers; 1996). The list has been customized to the particular needs of organizations working on reducing delays and waiting times.

Delays and Waiting Times

REDESIGN THE SYSTEM

1 Do Tasks in Parallel
2 Use Multiple Processes
3 Minimize Handoffs
4 Synchronize
5 Use Pull Systems
6 Move Steps Closer Together
7 Use Automation
8 Consider People to Be in the Same System
9 Use Multiple Processing Units
10 Extend the Time of Specialists
11 Convert Internal Steps to External

SHAPE THE DEMAND

12 Eliminate Things That Are Not Used
13 Insert an Informative Delay
14 Combine Services
15 Automate
16 Triage
17 Extinguish Demand for Ineffective Care
18 Relocate the Demand
19 Anticipate Demand
20 Promote Self-Care

MATCH CAPACITY TO DEMAND

21 Improve Predictions
22 Smooth the Work Flow
23 Adjust to Peak Demand
24 Identify and Manage the Constraint
25 Work Down the Backlog
26 Balance Centralized and Decentralized Capacity
27 Use Contingency Plans

Change Concepts Redesigning the

Products and services in all areas of the healthcare system are produced by processes. How does work flow in these processes? What is the plan to get work through a process? Are the various steps in the process arranged and prioritized to obtain quality outcomes at low cost and with minimum delay? How can we change the work flow so that the process is less reactive and more planned?

The following change concepts can help in analyzing and improving the flow of products and services through the healthcare system, resulting in significant reductions in delays and waiting times.

REDESIGN THE SYSTEM

1 Do Tasks in Parallel

2 Use Multiple Processes

3 Minimize Handoffs

4 Synchronize

5 Use Pull Systems

6 Move Steps Closer Together

7 Use Automation

8 Consider People to Be in the Same System

9 Use Multiple Processing Units

10 Extend the Time of Specialists

11 Convert Internal Steps to External

System

1 Do Tasks in Parallel

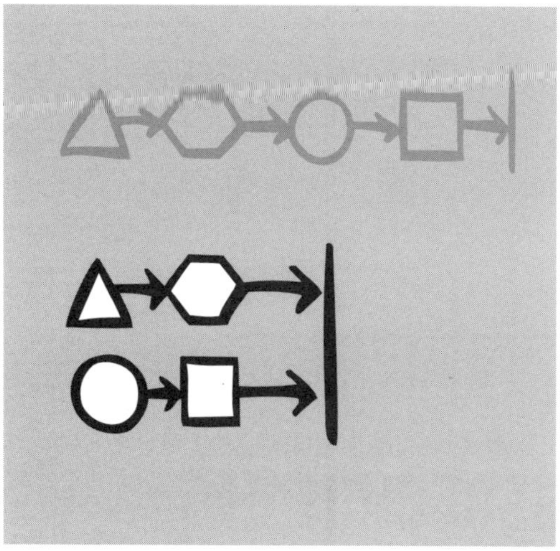

Instead of doing tasks sequentially, redesign the system to do some or all tasks in parallel.

Many systems are designed so that tasks are done in a series or a linear sequence. The second task is not begun until the first task is completed. This is especially true when different groups in the organization are involved in the different steps of a process. Sometimes improvements in time and cost can be gained from redesigning the system to do some or all tasks in parallel. For example, the work in step 5 can begin as soon as step 1 is complete, rather than waiting until steps 2, 3, and 4 are done.

EXAMPLES OF PROCESS CHANGES:

Prepare patient for surgery while setting up instruments.

The traditional surgical process for room set-up consists of three sequential steps: clean the floor and table, then set up the instruments, then prepare the patient. One hospital has increased its on-time starts for surgery by redesigning the process so that preparation of the patient and set-up of the instruments are done at the same time.

Obtain patient information during waiting times in course of treatment.

The first step for a patient being seen by a healthcare provider is usually a registration process in which the patient provides detailed clinical and reimbursement information before treatment begins. A quick admit process in the emergency department at several hospitals eliminates this delay. In this system, only basic information (e.g., name, payer source, and clinical complaint) is obtained from the patient before treatment; the remaining information is obtained throughout the course of treatment when the patient is not being seen by a provider. This same approach can be applied in the primary care office visit or clinic setting.

Begin discharge teaching during admit process.

Instead of waiting until the patient is clinically ready for discharge, several hospitals begin discharge teaching during the preadmit time prior to surgery, or as soon as the patient is admitted or diagnosed.

2 Use Multiple Processes

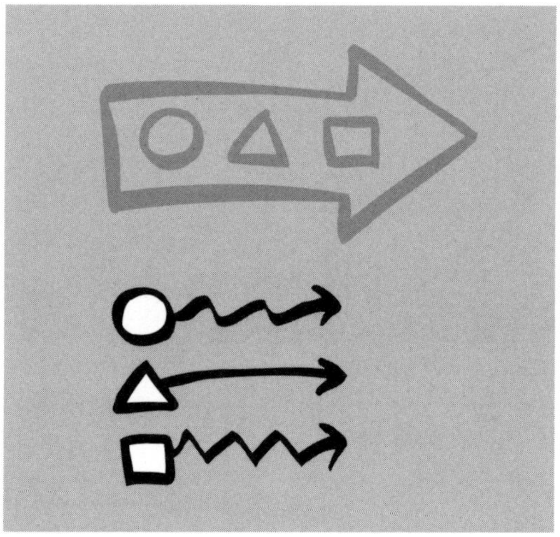

Rather than use a single "one size fits all" process, use multiple versions of the process, each tailored to the different needs of customers or users.

EXAMPLES OF PROCESS CHANGES:

Use separate processes for two classes of children's hospital patients.

A children's hospital cares for two broad classes of patients: "complex" and "acute but straightforward." The "complex" patients typically remain in the hospital for treatment lasting several days to several weeks. Many of the "acute but straightforward" patients stay in the hospital for 48 to 72 hours; some, less than 48 hours. Before their redesign, many of the processes used to care for the children were the same for both types of patients, even though they had very different needs. The processes have been redesigned so that different processes and services are used for the two types of patients. As a result, each type is better served and the length of stay for the acute care patients decreases significantly.

Use separate process for ED patients with less serious conditions.

Patients who are cared for in a hospital's emergency department vary in the complexity and seriousness of their conditions. Rather than having the same process for all types of patients, one hospital has created a separate process for patients with less serious conditions who can be treated more quickly and then released. ED staff identify charts for these patients at triage and move the patients through the care process as quickly as possible, while at the same time balancing the need to treat the critically ill or injured patients (often, a physician is able to treat one or two less serious patients while waiting for the test results on more complex, or more seriously ill, patients).

Use separate process for ED patients with extremity injuries.

Protocols to guide and standardize patient treatment can also be used to establish multiple processes for different types of patients. For example, even though emergency departments treat a number of different patient conditions, patients with extremity injuries constitute a category in need of similar types of tests and treatments, such as x-rays and stabilization of the injury. An ED team that establishes set protocols for the treatment of these patients can streamline care and reduce delays.

3 Minimize Handoffs

Redesign the work flow to minimize any handoffs in the process.

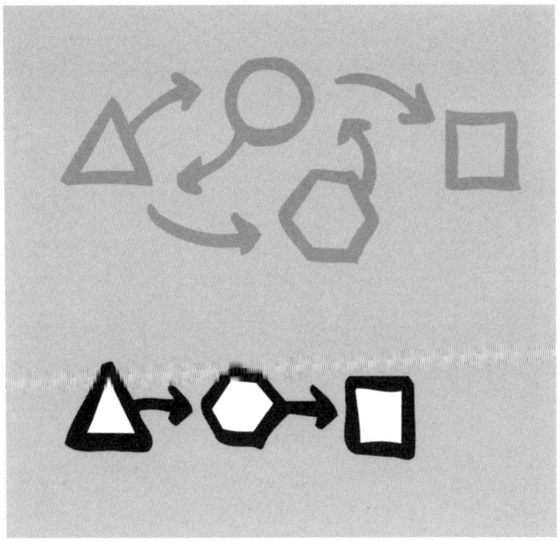

Many systems require that elements (e.g., a customer, a form, a product) be transferred to multiple people, offices, or work stations to complete the processing or service. The handoff from one stage to the next can incur increased time and costs and cause quality problems. It is often preferable to redesign the process so that fewer workers are involved in the process and any worker is involved only once per iteration of a process. For example, an organization can reduce layers of management that require multiple reviews, meetings, and approvals. It can expand clerical jobs to include scheduling, staffing, planning, and analysis. It can cross-train workers to handle many functions rather than being specialists in one specific function.

EXAMPLES OF PROCESS CHANGES:

Train the clinic receptionist to decide whether to schedule appointments.

Several HMOs and health systems have increased access to appointments for their patients by training the medical receptionist who takes calls from members to make the decision to schedule appointments. Before the training, the receptionist had to hand off the patient to a nurse who then decided whether an appointment was necessary. When this handoff is eliminated, the patient is able to get an appointment at the desired time with a minimum of delay, and the nurses have more time to provide care.

Have the same ED clinician perform various procedures.

In the emergency department in a children's hospital, the tasks of phlebotomy and IV insertion are performed by the same clinician.

Order x-rays at triage.

Before the process was redesigned, patients arriving in the emergency department with an extremity injury would go through triage, registration, rooming, nurse assessment, and physician evaluation before the physician would order x-rays. Under the redesigned process, patients are seen by the triage nurse upon arrival in the ED, the nurse orders x-rays as needed, x-rays are performed, and results are available at the time of physician evaluation.

4 Synchronize

Time all of the steps in a process with reference to a clearly defined, agreed-upon synchronization point.

Production of products and services usually involves multiple stages operating at different times and different speeds, resulting in an operation that is not coordinated. Much time can be spent waiting for another stage.

For example, in many ambulatory care clinics, providers, staff, and patients have different understandings of what an "8 AM appointment" means. If the registration desk doesn't open until 8 AM, there is no way the patient can be placed in a room, have his history taken, and be ready to see the physician at 8 AM. If all agree that "8 AM appointment" means "Physician sees patient at 8 AM," then tasks can be synchronized around that point and waiting times can be reduced.

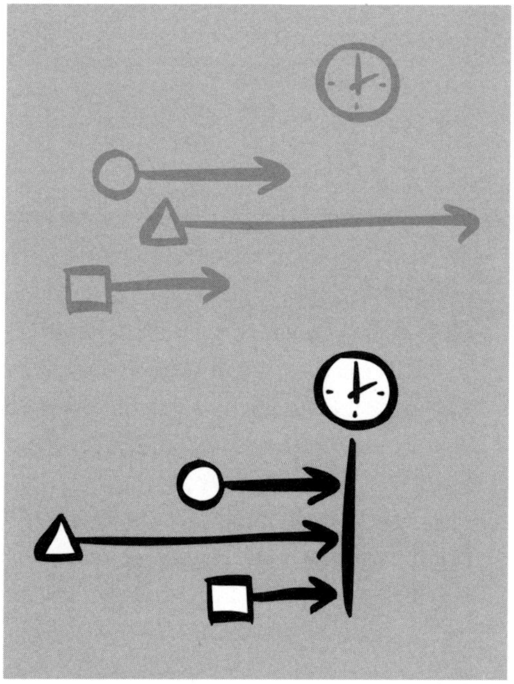

EXAMPLES OF PROCESS CHANGES:

Make synchronization point for surgery the incision time.

A hospital uses "incision time for surgery" as the synchronization point for all of the processes leading up to the actual surgery itself, including patient registration, pre-anesthesia preparation, room set-up and anesthesia. Once the synchronization point is defined and agreed on, all processes can be timed with reference to that point.

Make synchronization point for ambulatory care the moment when the physician walks into the examining room.

Many processes must be streamlined and coordinated to reduce delays for the patient at this synchronization point, including registration, location of patient charts, availability of results of lab tests and x-rays, patient education, patient history, preventive services, and escorting the patient to the exam room. Delays can be reduced by drastically shortening the patient registration step in the office visit process; the patient is escorted directly into the exam room, rather than waiting in the waiting room.

5 Use Pull Systems

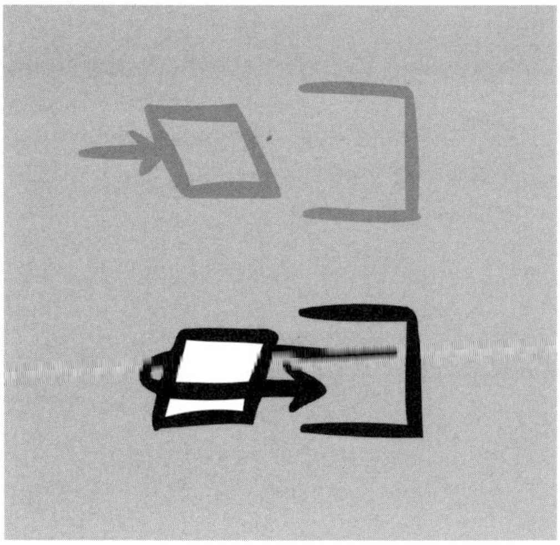

When work is being transferred through a process, instead of "pushing" it from one step to the next, have the later step "pull" it from the previous step.

In a pull system of service, the timely transition of work from one step in the process to another is the primary responsibility of the downstream (i.e., subsequent) process—for example, the ICU orchestrating the transfer of the patient from the emergency department. This is in contrast to most traditional "push systems," in which the transition of work is the responsibility of the upstream (i.e., prior) process—for example, the emergency department trying to "push" patients into the ICU.

Pull systems can be created whenever a patient is being moved from one point of care to the next. This is particularly important when the patient is being transferred from one care setting to another. Smooth communication and cooperation are keys to pull systems for patient transfer.

EXAMPLES OF PROCESS CHANGES:

Pull patients from ED to inpatient unit.

The Be-a-Bed-Ahead system addresses the delay in moving patients from one point of care to the next, for example, from the emergency department to the inpatient unit or to the intensive care unit (ICU). Before redesign, delays occurred between the time when the ED staff notified the inpatient unit that a patient needed a bed and the time the patient was actually transferred. The call from the ED to the floor triggered a chain of events that eventually led to the patient's being moved to the inpatient unit. In contrast, under the Be-a-Bed-Ahead system the inpatient units anticipates the demand (by measuring demand over time) and has a bed ready into which a patient can be moved ("pulled" rather than "pushed") as soon as the demand occurs.

Pull asthma patients from ED to primary care site.

Before redesign of emergency asthma treatment, asthma patients seen in the emergency department were often told to make an appointment at a primary care site for follow-up care. However, many patients never made that appointment. In the redesigned system, the primary care clinic established a pull system by having slots available so that the staff in the ED can make the appointment for the patient before the patient leaves the ED. In this way, the primary care site is pulling the patient into its scheduling system rather than waiting for the patient to call to request an appointment or show up later, unannounced, with an urgent situation.

6 Move Steps Closer Together

Move the physical location of adjacent steps in a process close together so that work can be passed directly from one step to the next.

The physical location of people and facilities can affect process time and cause communication problems. Moving steps close together eliminates the need for communication systems (such as mail) and physical transports (such as supply and pharmacy delivery systems). If it is not possible to move steps in a process closer, consider electronic hookups. For some processes, computer networks with common file structures can have an effect similar to moving the steps physically closer.

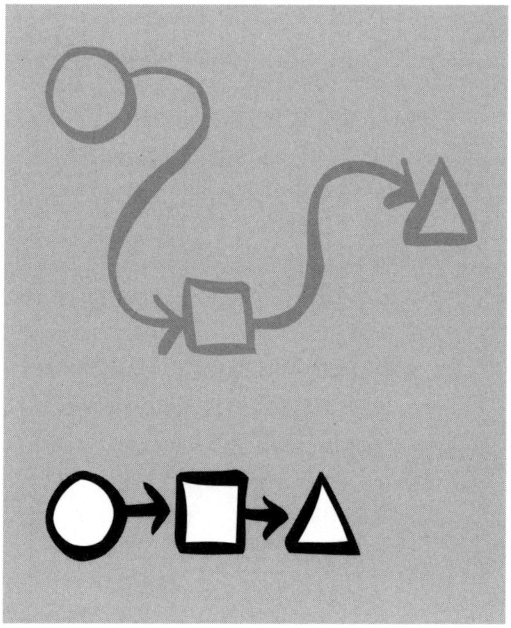

EXAMPLES OF PROCESS CHANGES:

Move radiography suite next to ED.

To eliminate delays in obtaining diagnostic testing for ED patients, one hospital has moved its radiography suite next to the emergency department.

Move outpatient surgery (OPS) support to OPS area.

Another hospital has relocated all departments providing support for outpatient surgery directly in the OPS area.

Move patient's chart to the bedside.

One hospital has relocated the patient's chart to the bedside, instead of having portions of the medical record in many different locations.

7 Use Automation

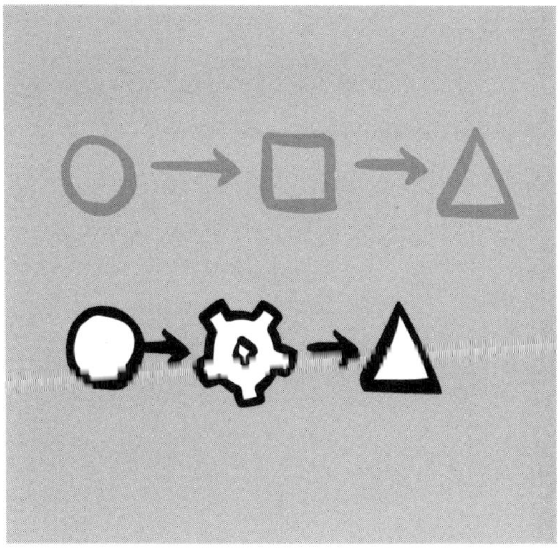

Improve the flow of processes by the intelligent use of automation.

Consider automation to improve the work flow for any process to reduce costs, reduce cycle times, eliminate human slips, reduce repetitive manual tasks, and provide measurement.

EXAMPLES OF PROCESS CHANGES:

Use hand-held computers in preop testing.

One hospital uses automation creatively to reduce delays in preoperative testing for surgery patients. A patient uses a hand-held computer, prompting answers to questions that assess the patient's need for different levels of preoperative testing. Patients with low risk levels may not need the full complement of tests, and in some cases may be able to report directly to the hospital or surgical center on the day of surgery, rather than being scheduled for a separate preadmission testing regimen.

Use faxes to notify nurses on receiving units.

Automation can also be used to facilitate the movement of patients from one point of care to the next. One hospital uses faxes to notify nurses on the receiving units that a patient is being moved from another area of the hospital. Similarly, units use faxes to communicate bed availability to a central depot for information.

8 Consider People to Be in the Same System

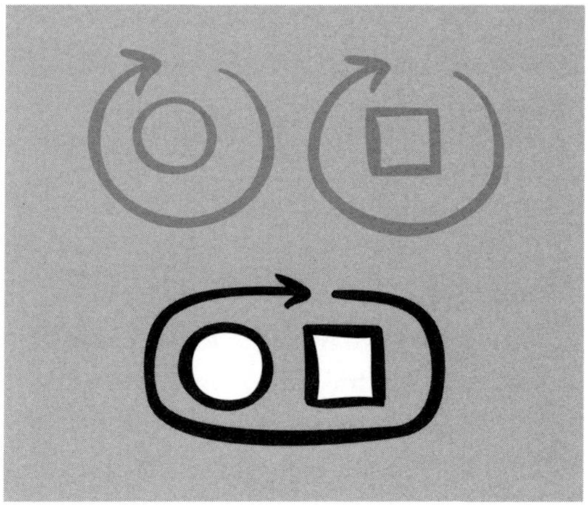

Take steps to help people see themselves as part of the same system working toward common goals.

Giving individuals a common purpose provides a basis for optimizing the larger system instead of each unit trying to optimize its own system.

EXAMPLES OF PROCESS CHANGES:

Consider surgeon's office and hospital as parts of same system.

Reducing surgical delays requires balancing the needs and interests of the surgeons and the hospital, and finding solutions that maximize the ability of the system to function efficiently. For example, not everyone can have the most popular start times for surgery, so physicians must be flexible. At the same time, physicians' offices have an interest in streamlining the scheduling process for surgery as well as for preadmission testing. The hospital can develop processes that reduce delays and rework for office staff such as providing physicians' offices with access to computerized scheduling or directions to the hospital for distribution to their patients.

See all processes leading to surgery as parts of same system.

The successful use of synchronization as a change concept (see 4: Synchronize) involves getting people to see themselves as part of the same system. For example, synchronizing all the steps needed to start a surgery on time requires everyone in the surgery process to agree that the incision point is the key reference point for the process—and then to adjust all the steps leading to that point so that the surgery can begin without delays.

Consider ED and floor nurses as parts of same system.

Establishing a pull system (see Change Concept 5: Use Pull Systems) also requires a systems view. For example, nurses on the floor who redesign their system to have a bed always ready for a patient being transferred from the ED understand that the entire system in the hospital is geared toward moving the patient from one unit to another in the hospital without delays.

Consider x-ray, lab, and ED as parts of same system.

One hospital helps the staff understand the effect of x-ray and lab turnaround time on emergency department delays by posting run charts in the other departments showing ED delays.

9 Use Multiple Processing Units

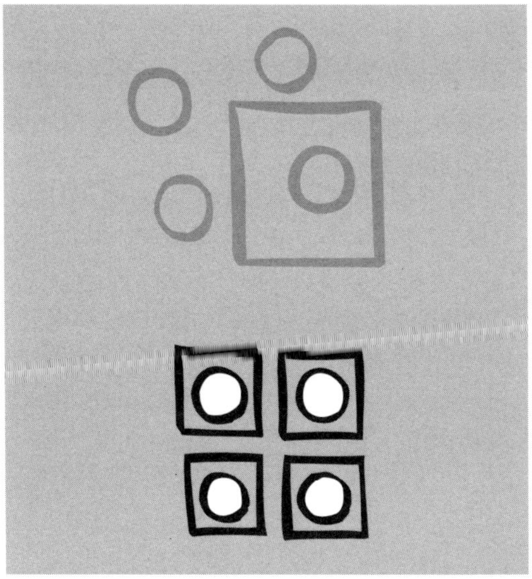

To gain flexibility in controlling the flow of work, try to have multiple work stations, equipment, or processes in a system—all of the same type.

This makes it possible to run smaller lots, service special customers, minimize the impact of maintenance and down-time, and add flexibility to staffing.

EXAMPLES OF PROCESS CHANGES:

Use several small centrifuges instead of one large centrifuge.

Before redesign, a hospital used one large centrifuge for blood analysis but found that delays occurred since the lab staff had to wait until the centrifuge was full before running the tests. Using multiple processing units (e.g., having several small centrifuges) allows for continual blood testing since the small machines are run more often.

Designate an alternate site for sub-specialty patients.

To meet the need for an inpatient sub-specialty bed when none is available, one hospital has designated a second site where staff are cross-trained to care for those "specialized" patients.

Use identical room set-ups for surgery.

In surgery, delays often occur when the patient and the surgical team are ready for surgery, but the assigned room is still being used for the previous surgery. Additional surgical suites are available, but the room set-up is not appropriate for the type of surgery to be performed. Using identical room set-ups for as many surgical rooms as possible provides greater flexibility for meeting scheduled as well as unexpected demand.

10 Extend the Time of Specialists

Have specialists do only the tasks that require their specific skills.

Most organizations employ specialists who have specific skills or knowledge, but not all of their work duties require the use of these skills or knowledge. Try to remove assignments and job requirements that do not utilize the specialists' skills, or find ways to let the specialists have a broader impact on the organization. This is especially important if the specialists are a constraint to throughput in the system.

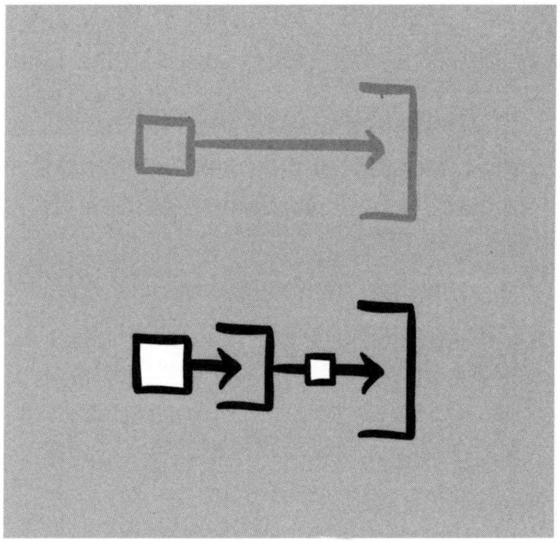

EXAMPLE OF PROCESS CHANGES:

Use skills and expertise of each member of the primary care team.

This change is central to several organizations' efforts to reduce delays in the office setting. Changes made include the following: Receptionists are trained to schedule patients automatically for the appropriate type of appointment, rather than handing off that function to a nurse. Nurses now review patient charts before the patient is seen by the physician, to identify educational or preventive services that could be provided by a nurse and to identify tests needed to support physician examination and treatment. Physician assistants are used in some settings to provide routine clinical care.

Use video and information technology to extend specialists' time.

Several organizations use videos for patient education. Videos convey information clearly and consistently—and they free physicians for tasks that require their specific skills.

11 Convert Internal Steps to External

Convert tasks that are done as part of the process to tasks that are performed ahead of time or deferred until later.

This is what is meant by converting a step to be external to the process. This conversion includes tasks that can be made external simply by redefining the time at which they are performed as well as tasks that can be made external only after some change is made to the process, such as new training or an improved information system.

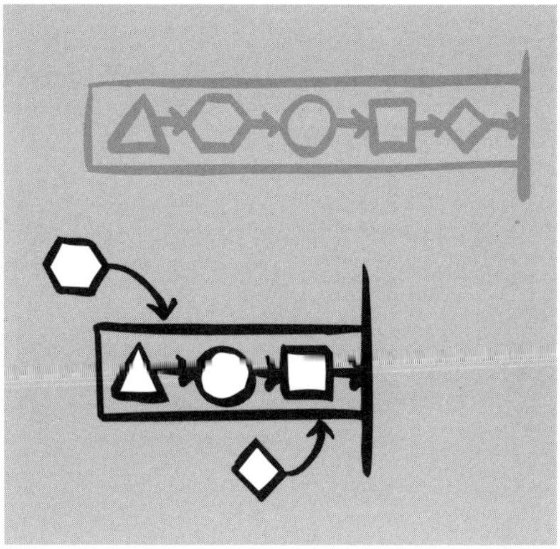

EXAMPLES OF PROCESS CHANGES:

Have standardized doses available ahead of time.

A hospital wants to reduce the time it takes to get a medication to a patient unit. By studying the needs of similar patients, the team can standardize doses for some frequently used medications. This allows the medications to be made up in advance of the request (i.e., external to the system) and significantly reduces the delays.

Move consultations from ED to inpatient setting.

When the decision is made to admit a patient from the emergency department, one hospital moves consultations from the ED to the inpatient setting if they are not necessary for initiating treatment or for making the decision to admit.

Customize central supplies for particular physicians.

A surgical service reduced delays in room set-up by customizing certain physicians' supplies. Previously, central supply would provide a surgical cart with most of the supplies needed for a particular type of surgery. However, surgical support staff would then have to find additional supplies that were needed for particular physicians. This led to delays in surgery set-up. Now central supply has a list of the supplies requested by each physician and can provide the customized set-up along with the standard supplies.

Change Concepts Shaping Demand

Much of health care is delivered according to habits and beliefs that could safely, if not easily, be changed. Conversations about patient expectations or educating patients often focus on opportunities for influencing the demand for care, with the intent of reducing costs, improving outcomes, or both. However, actual efforts to reshape demand are remarkably few, and often rely simply on blunt disincentives (like copayment) or barriers (like gatekeeping or queues). Many sound change concepts await an organization that wishes to reduce delays and waiting times by reshaping the demand for care.

SHAPE THE DEMAND

12 Eliminate Things That Are Not Used

13 Insert an Informative Delay

14 Combine Services

15 Automate

16 Triage

17 Extinguish Demand for Ineffective Care

18 Relocate the Demand

19 Anticipate Demand

20 Promote Self-Care

12 Eliminate Things That Are Not Used

Cease to supply something not wanted or rarely used.

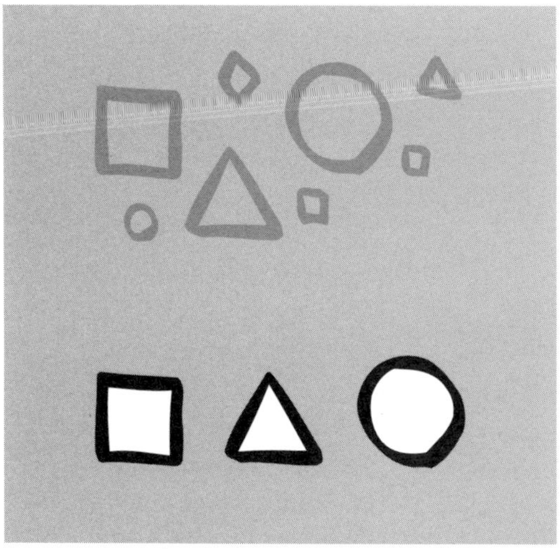

EXAMPLE OF PROCESS CHANGE:

Eliminate drugs that are seldom used.

The use of hospital formularies eliminates drugs that are seldom used. For example, instead of having a choice of 20 types of antibiotics, physicians can choose from a list of 10 that provide the same clinical effect. This reduces the number of drugs the pharmacy has to stock, simplifies the ordering of drugs, and reduces delays in filling the physician's order.

13 Insert an Informative Delay

Postpone immediate service for the specific purpose of obtaining information from the waiting period.

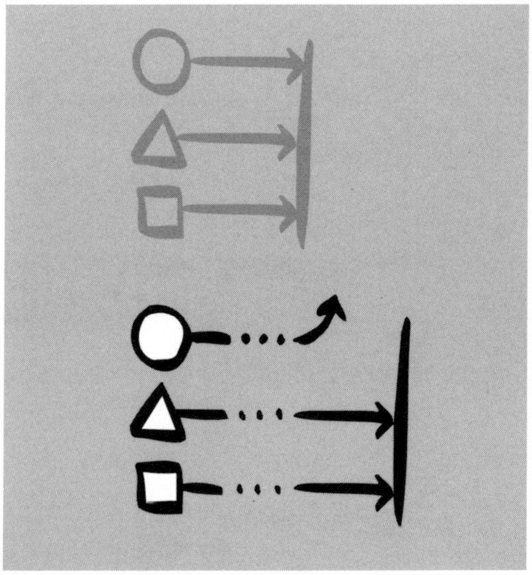

EXAMPLES OF PROCESS CHANGES:

Wait for conditions to improve with time.

The parent of a toddler requests an appointment to have the febrile child examined. The nurse practitioner predicts that the child's upper respiratory infection should improve within two days and suggests that the parent bring him in after two days if he is not improved. This triaging of patient phone calls can be done in a way that doesn't appear to the patient (or parent) as a barrier to care, but as a way of providing care when appropriate and needed.

Educate patients during waiting times.

Another type of informative delay involves using waiting times during the office visit to conduct patient education. This might occur in the waiting room or even in the exam room. Although the goal is to reduce these waiting times, effective patient education can be interspersed throughout the patient visit.

14 Combine Services

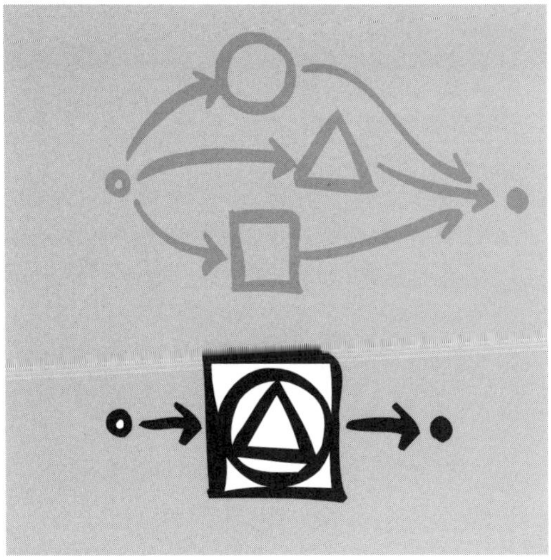

Reframe the original demand for individualized service into a larger cluster of services.

The combined services will be easier for the producer to satisfy and often more effective for the patient ("We can give you not only A but also B.").

EXAMPLE OF PROCESS CHANGE:

Group appointments for patients with hypertension.

Demand for primary care appointments for routine monitoring of chronic conditions often contributes to delays in other patients' being able to get timely appointments. One HMO identified hypertensive patients as high users of office appointments and determined that the level of care provided to patients with hypertension in individual appointments could be provided equally well in group appointments, where routine checks on blood pressure as well as ongoing patient education could be conducted. This not only contributes to reducing demand on the appointment calendar; it also provides a more socially supportive atmosphere for the patients.

15 Automate

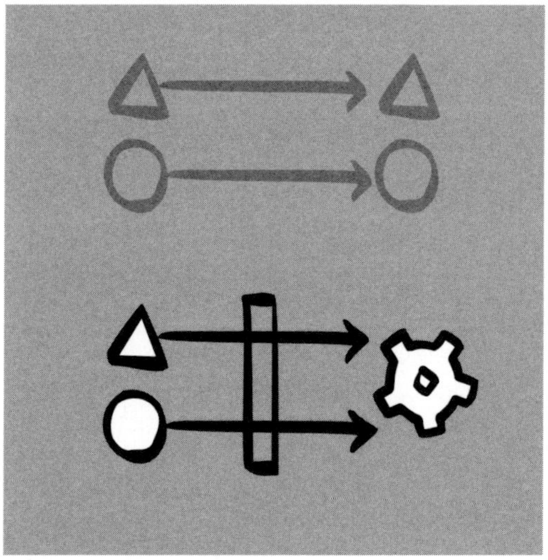

Meet a recurrent need with a standardized process.

Reframe the original request for an individualized service to one for which you have a standardized product ("That's a request of type Z, and we have a special way to help you.").

EXAMPLE OF PROCESS CHANGE:

Answer clinical questions via audiotape.

An HMO has established a library of short, prerecorded audiotapes with answers to 200 frequently asked clinical questions (e.g., What are the symptoms of gonorrhea? How do you contract AIDS? Where can I find out what immunizations I need for travel to Africa? What can I do if my baby has colic?). Switchboard operators are trained to listen to callers' questions, to offer them a chance to hear the relevant tape recording, and then to ask if they need further assistance.

16 Triage

Establish multiple channels for satisfying different needs that originally present as the same.

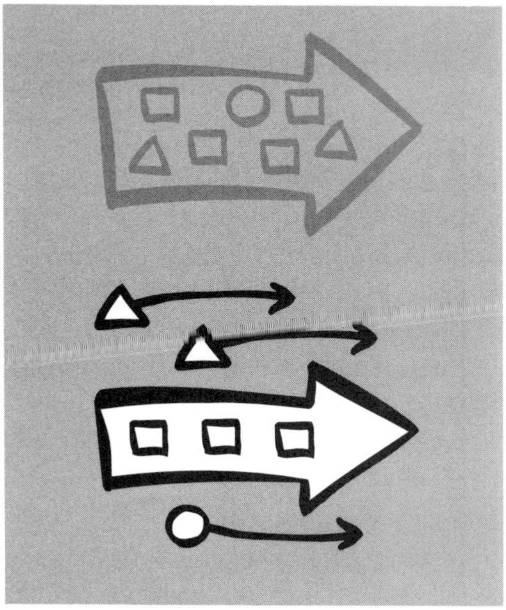

EXAMPLES OF PROCESS CHANGES:

Refer patients directly to specialists.

An HMO that formerly required a gatekeeping primary care visit before a referral to dermatology analyzes its experience and determines that a certain subset of requests always results in a referral. It eliminates gatekeeping for that subset, and directly refers patients who call for primary care visits for skin conditions.

Have a separate system in ED for nonemergent conditions.

An emergency department develops a separate Med Express system to identify and treat patients with non-emergent, uncomplicated illnesses and injuries.

17 Extinguish Demand for Ineffective Care

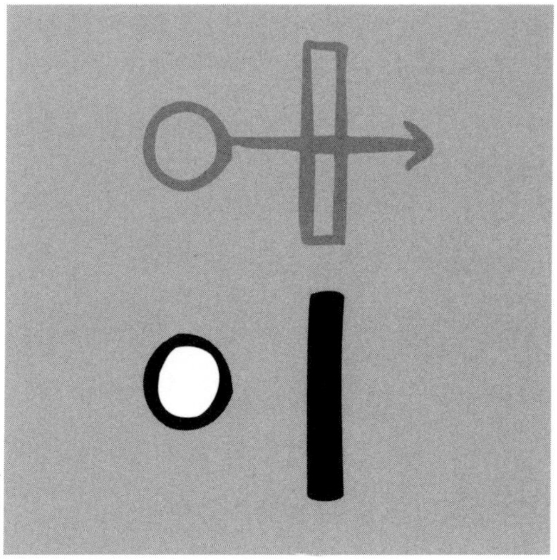

Do not provide care for which there is no evidence of efficacy.

A great deal of health care has little or no scientific foundation, and some care used regularly is actually known to be harmful. Few healthcare organizations appear to have become adept at directing patients' expectations away from unnecessary or harmful care. This is fertile terrain for process innovation.

EXAMPLES OF PROCESS CHANGES:

Minimize treatment that has no evidence of efficacy.

In its *Guide to Clinical Preventive Services*, the U.S. Preventive Services Task Force reports on over 200 commonly performed preventive practices, and finds a lack of scientific foundation for many of them. An HMO adopts the task force guidelines for effective prevention, and conducts a wide-ranging literature campaign for its enrollees and caregivers. (See U.S. Preventive Services Task Force. *Guide to Clinical Preventive Services*. 2nd ed. Baltimore, MD: Williams & Wilkins; 1996.)

Allow longer intervals between camp physicals.

A managed care association works with the state public health department to extend the recency requirement for routine camp physical examinations from one year to two years prior to the start of a camp session.

18 Relocate the Demand

Meet the demand for a service, but in a different location from where it is originally requested ("You get that there, not here.").

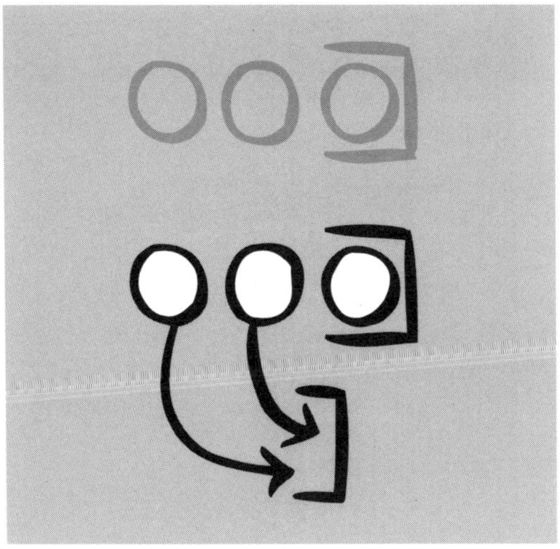

EXAMPLES OF PROCESS CHANGES:

Administer immunizations in school.

In a small city, pediatricians work with the school and public health departments to arrange for all immunizations for children over four years of age to be administered in schools.

Have LPN remove sutures.

A group practice explains to patients whose lacerations are sutured that sutures are routinely removed by a well-trained LPN.

Schedule lunch hour check-ups.

A busy primary care practice offers its downtown patients the chance to be seen for a check-up during their lunch hour, so long as the patients do not require that the visit be with their usual primary care doctor. Some patients prefer the convenience to the continuity, others prefer the reverse.

19 Anticipate Demand

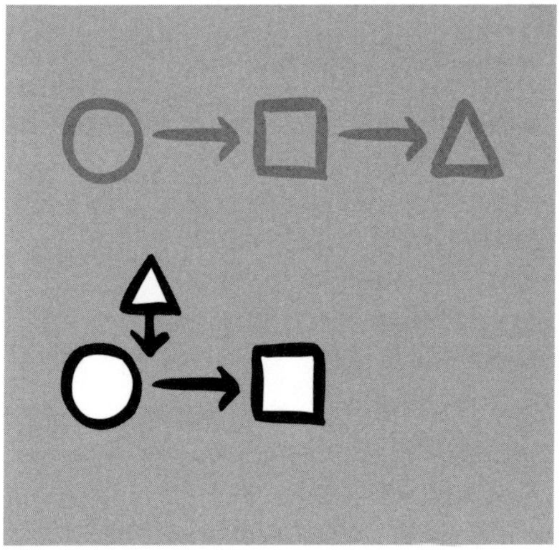

Meet a need before it arises.

The caregiver predicts that a need will develop and, instead of waiting, meets the need, often at a time and place more convenient for both the caregiver and the patient ("You don't know yet that you will need this, but you probably will, so here it is.").

EXAMPLES OF PROCESS CHANGES:

Give breast-feeding instruction prior to discharge.

An obstetrical service has a breast-feeding instructor who visits the mother routinely prior to discharge. This costs the hospital a little more during the short hospital stay, but saves several times as much in fewer phone calls and visits for breast-feeding problems in subsequent weeks.

Have cardiac nurse visit patient at home preoperatively.

A hospital sends a cardiac nurse into the home of every open heart patient preoperatively to describe what will happen during and after surgery, to set up home rehabilitation, and to recommend physical adaptations in home equipment and layout. This program reduces the length of stay by two full days, improves patient satisfaction, and hastens the patient's return to work.

20 Promote Self-Care

Create or reveal the capacity of patients to treat themselves ("You don't need us to do that; you can do it yourself.").

This is probably the most powerful of all change concepts in shaping demand, yet it still remains to be explored in process changes in real healthcare settings.

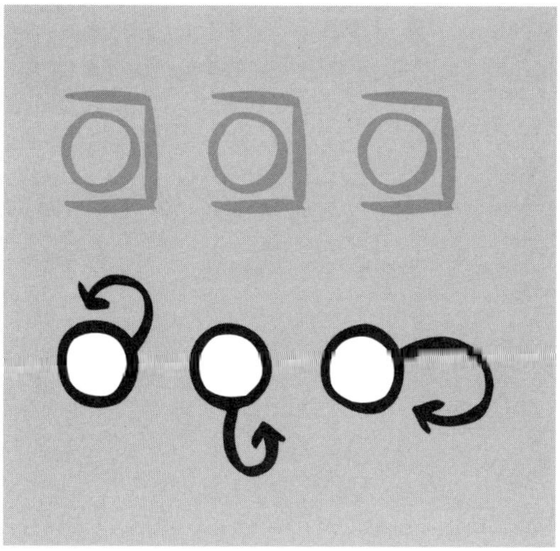

EXAMPLES OF PROCESS CHANGES:

Provide nebulizer therapy at home.

Children with asthma receive nebulizer therapy from their parents using a machine in the home. Parents maintain run charts of peak expiratory flow, and they implement decision rules about initiation of second-tier and third-tier medications.

Use diagnostic testing at home.

Home pregnancy testing kits are available in grocery stores.

Teach in-home otoscope use.

A pediatrician trains mothers of children with frequent ear infections to use an otoscope at home and to phone in their descriptions rather than visit the office.

Change Concepts Matching Capacity

Sometimes minor adjustments in the availability of the healthcare provider or the scheduling of patient appointments are sufficient to reduce delays. Whenever a quantitative analysis indicates that the system has the capacity to meet the demand during normal functioning, then specific change concepts can be implemented relatively quickly to help align capacity and demand during predicted or unpredicted periods of high demand. Accomplishing this requires flexibility in the system, willingness of staff to see themselves as part of the same system, and the ability of the system to make adjustments to meet the immediate demand.

MATCH CAPACITY TO DEMAND

21 Improve Predictions
22 Smooth the Work Flow
23 Adjust to Peak Demand
24 Identify and Manage the Constraint
25 Work Down the Backlog
26 Balance Centralized and Decentralized Capacity
27 Use Contingency Plans

to Demand

21 Improve Predictions

Predict demand based on past experience and plan capacity to meet predictions.

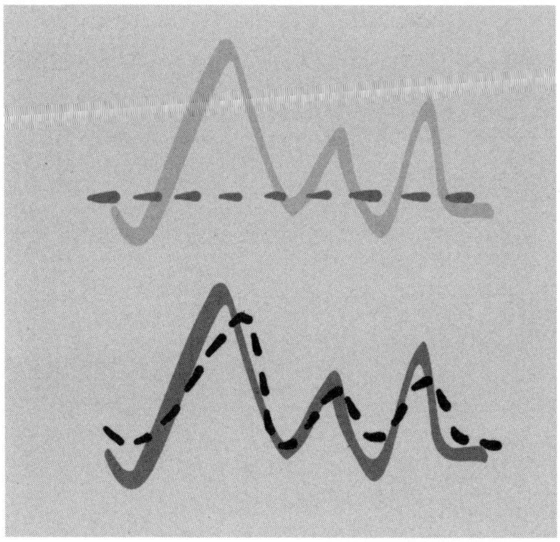

Plans, resources, and staffing are based on predictions. For many situations, predictions are built from the ground up each time a prediction is required; historical data are not used. The study of variation from past experience can lead to alternative ways to improve the predictions. Healthcare organizations can use the following approaches to develop predictions of demand: use leading indicators (e.g., early indications of a particularly severe flu season), anticipate special causes (e.g., ED preparing for heart attacks and sprains after a heavy snowfall), use simple averages of historical data (e.g., average number of requests for same-day appointments in primary care), and use regression models (e.g., relate patient demographics to frequency of specialty appointments).

EXAMPLES OF PROCESS CHANGES:

Predict periods of high ED demand.

An emergency department tracks demand in order to identify the days of the week, and hours of the day, when demand is especially high. The ED is now able to predict periods of high demand and make system adjustments (for example, moving staff from low-demand periods to high-demand periods) to meet these conditions.

Use predictions of demand to set panel sizes and staffing.

An HMO is able to predict the number of visits per year per thousand patients in its covered population. On the basis of this prediction, it is able to make plans to meet the demand with appropriate panel sizes and staffing. (See Smoller M. Telephone calls and appointment requests. Predictability in an unpredictable world. *HMO Pract.* 1992;6(2):25–29.)

Predict demand for same-day appointments.

Office practices study the demand for appointments with primary care physicians. As a result, they set aside from 30% to 70% of their appointments for same-day appointments. The number of canceled appointments drops dramatically, patient satisfaction increases, and productivity improves.

22 Smooth the Work Flow

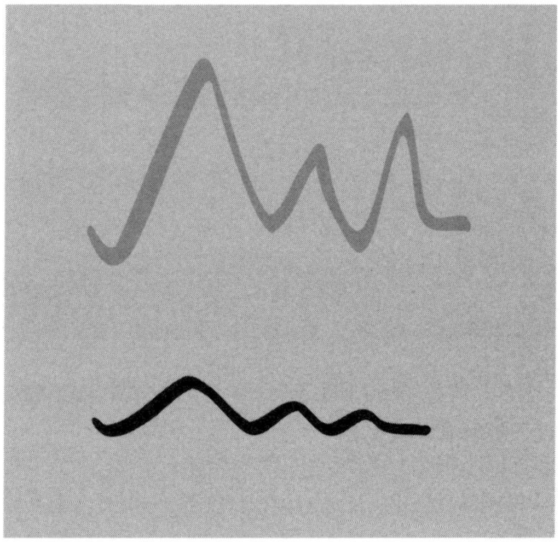

Take steps to reduce fluctuations in demand.

Changes in demand often cause work flow to fluctuate widely at different times of the year, month, week, or day. Rather than trying to increase staff to handle the peak demands, managers can often take steps to better distribute the demand. This results in a smooth work flow rather than continual peaks and valleys.

EXAMPLES OF PROCESS CHANGES:

Schedule routine care at low-demand times.

Scheduling can often be used to smooth the work flow. One primary care clinic solicits appointments for routine care such as mammography testing, anticipating demand and fitting patients into low-demand time slots.

Intersperse variable-length appointments throughout the day.

Anticipating the duration of clinic visits of various types is another method of smoothing the work flow. Several clinics now take into account both physician and patient preferences, establishing a small number of appointment types and durations that can be used for standard scheduling.

23 Adjust to Peak Demand

If fluctuations in demand cannot be reduced further, make plans to meet periods of high demand.

Sometimes it is not possible to shape the demand on a system or match the demand to the system capacity. In these cases, instead of keeping a fixed amount of resources (e.g., supplies, rooms, clinicians), managers can use historical data to predict peak demand periods. Then temporary methods to meet the demand can be implemented (e.g., adding capacity during periods of predictably high demand).

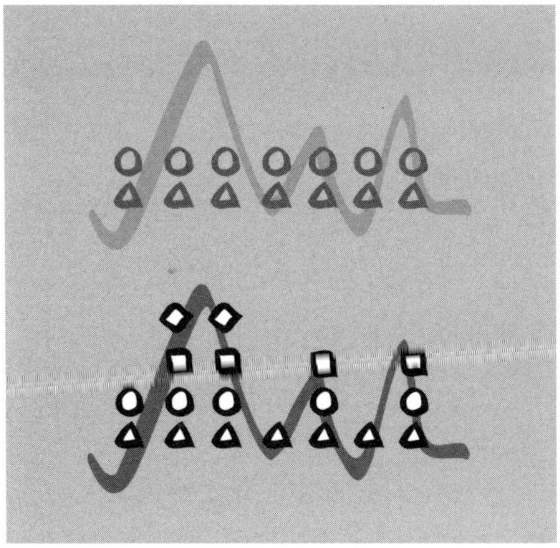

EXAMPLES OF PROCESS CHANGES:

Match physicians' schedules with patient demand.

Scheduling to meet demand is often key to reducing delays for patients. For example, if Monday morning is a high-demand time for primary care, but additional physicians are not scheduled for appointments during those times, then patients will either experience delays or access to the service will be compromised. One HMO analyzed peak demand times and then worked with physicians to create more flexible scheduling. Physicians are now available for evening or early morning hours to match patient demand for these appointment times. In addition, a "physician of the day" is assigned to remain in the office until all patients have been seen on that particular day.

Adjust ED staff to periods of predictably high demand.

Long waiting lines develop in an emergency department on Friday nights, and the ED adjusts its staff to accommodate this time of predictably high demand.

24 Identify and Manage the Constraint

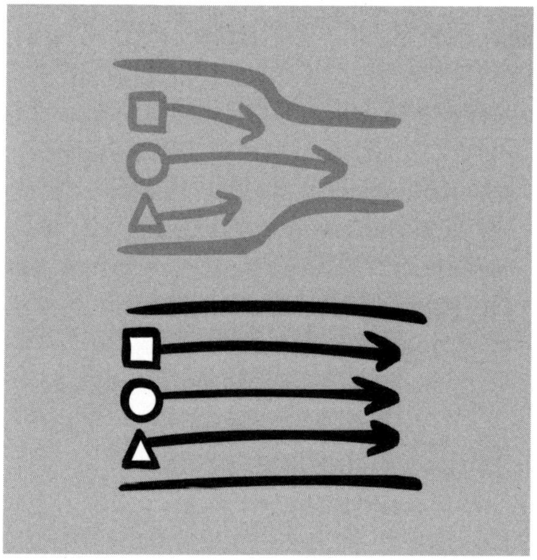

Find and remove the bottlenecks in the system.

A bottleneck or constraint is anything that restricts the throughput of a system. A constraint within an organization is any resource for which the demand is greater than its available capacity. In order to increase the throughput in a system, the constraints must be identified, exploited if possible, and removed if necessary. Bottlenecks occur in many parts of life: exits to a concert hall, rush hour traffic, the telephone receptionist, the cashier in a cafeteria line. They can usually be found by looking where people are waiting or where work is piling up.

EXAMPLES OF PROCESS CHANGES:

Use physicians' time wisely.

Physicians at an HMO provide unscheduled routine care (such as immunizations) to scheduled patients when time permits. This maximizes the services of the physician and also works to reduce future demand on the system by anticipating the demand for the immunization that would be made at a future time.

Make all operating rooms available.

A bottleneck can also be a room or a piece of equipment. For example, one hospital standardizes the equipment and supplies available in each operating room, to eliminate delays in the surgery process that used to occur while operating rooms were being set up with equipment needed for specific cases. A group practice applies the same principle to standardizing the supplies that are stocked in its examination rooms at its primary care clinics (see Change Concept 9: Use Multiple Processing Units).

Free up ED exam rooms.

An emergency department finds that its doctors and nurses are waiting for exam rooms to become available in order to see patients. They establish an "asthma chair." Instead of tying up an exam room, patients are immediately triaged to the "chair," where treatment is begun using a protocol.

25 Work Down the Backlog

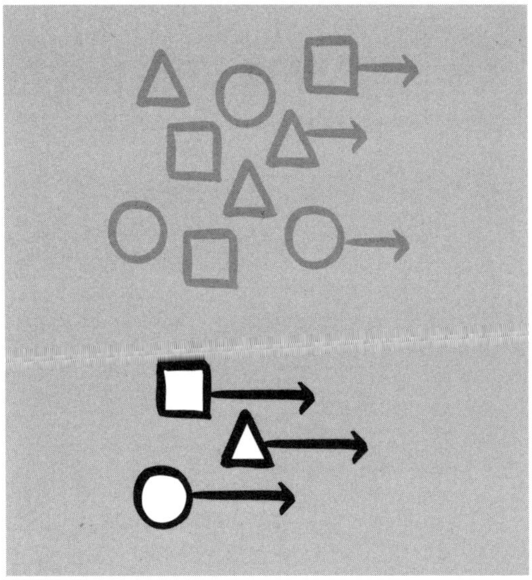

If a system has accumulated a backlog, add some capacity in the short term to reduce the backlog.

Unless the backlog is eliminated, the system will continue to carry this burden, marring any new steps that are taken to redesign the system. (See Part 4, for detailed instructions for working down the backlog.)

EXAMPLES OF PROCESS CHANGES:

Take on additional work in the short term.

One clinic reduces its backlog gradually by having physicians conduct one extra physical per week and having staff work one extra Saturday per month over a three-month period.

Use additional providers in the short term.

One clinic brings in additional providers temporarily to help reduce its backlog.

26 Balance Centralized and Decentralized Capacity

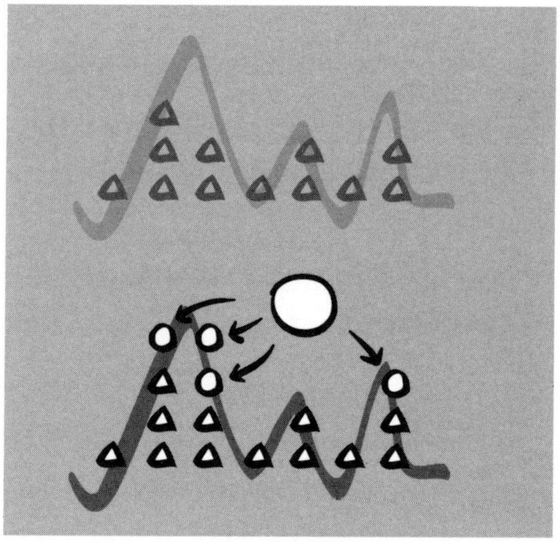

Use centralized staff to meet fluctuations in demand at the local level.

Hospitals and clinics often find it is efficient to centralize staff for some functions, yet there are clear advantages to decentralized staffing as well. Developing a plan that balances the two is a challenge. In general, it is advisable to make gross adjustments locally; that is, have enough local capacity to meet the average demand. Then make fine adjustments centrally; that is, draw on centralized staff to "top off" as local demand varies.

EXAMPLES OF PROCESS CHANGES:

Use centralized staff in high-demand periods.

In one hospital, the ICU has enough respiratory therapists on staff to meet the average demand. However, when demand for respiratory therapy exceeds the capacity on the ICU, the unit can draw on the centralized staff temporarily for extra help.

Cross-train centralized staff.

One hospital attempts to match nursing/patient ratios in the face of a fluctuating census. In addition to having each of 20 nursing units establish its own local staffing pattern, the hospital has a central staff of cross-trained nurses available to fill in when needed.

27 Use Contingency Plans

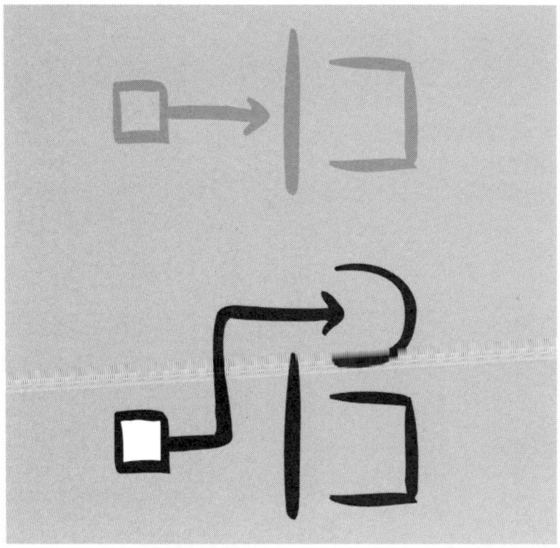

Prepare backup plans, or contingencies, to deal with unexpected delays.

The natural variation that occurs as part of the everyday functioning of a healthcare organization often creates problems. Reducing the variation might eventually reduce the problems, but how do people cope in the meantime? One way is to prepare backup plans to deal with unexpected situations. Cross-training is an important way to prepare for contingency planning because it enables staff to assume different duties as needed.

EXAMPLES OF PROCESS CHANGES:

Prepare a contingency plan when the physician is called to ED.

The staff of a doctor's office develops a contingency plan for those times when the doctor is called to the ED: the receptionist immediately notifies all patients in the waiting room and offers to reschedule. In addition, the receptionist calls all the patients who are scheduled for later appointments and offers to reschedule or to allow them to wait at home for a call notifying them when the doctor is again available.

Cross-train ED staff to meet shifting demand.

In an emergency department, staff are cross-trained so that they can fill in when there is temporarily high demand. For example, the respiratory therapist is also trained as an x-ray technician; nurses are also trained to do the work of phlebotomists.

THUS FAR IN THE GUIDE, YOU HAVE LEARNED:

Part 1

The Model for Improvement that can be applied to any area you want to improve.

Part 2

A step-by-step guide to using that model to work on reducing delays and waiting times, with each of the basic steps—setting aims, forming the team, establishing measures, and developing and testing changes—illustrated with examples.

Part 3

Three strategies for reducing delays and waiting times—redesign the system, shape demand, and match capacity to demand—and for each strategy, a group of change concepts to use as a starting point for generating good ideas for changes.

Part 4

Achieving Breakthrough Improvement in Four Key Areas

This section provides a comprehensive guide—a preplanned "guided tour"—to reducing delays and waiting times in four key areas.

Achieving Breakthrough Improvement

The organizations in the Breakthrough Series Collaborative focused their efforts on reducing delays and waiting times in four areas; the information in this section is based on the changes they made and the lessons they learned in the course of their work.

REDUCING DELAYS IN SURGERY

REDUCING DELAYS IN THE EMERGENCY DEPARTMENT

REDUCING DELAYS IN CLINICS AND PHYSICIANS' OFFICES

INCREASING ACCESS TO CARE

This section describes the major obstacles that organizations encountered, the changes that they tested to overcome the obstacles, and the measures they used to tell whether the changes were leading to improvement.

in Four Key Areas

EACH OF THE FOUR AREAS INCLUDES THE FOLLOWING:

The major obstacles to reducing delays and waiting times

The major obstacles, or difficult systems issues, that organizations needed to overcome in order to make progress.

Changes to overcome the obstacle

For each of the major obstacles identified, a detailed description of several process changes developed and tested by organizations that were found to be effective in reducing delays and waiting times. In many cases, the change concepts used to develop process changes are noted.

Measures that have proven useful

For each area, two sets of measures:

Standard measures that indicate whether changes that are made lead to improvement.

Balancing measures to make sure that changes made to improve one part of the system do not adversely affect other parts of the system.

For both sets of measures, instructions on what to measure and how to measure it.

Of course, organizations need not be limited to addressing these obstacles, trying the changes suggested to overcome the obstacles, or using these measures. They are meant only as a starting point. The particular issues of each system of care may well determine which obstacles to address, which changes to try, or which measures to collect. The sum total of all of these changes, however, begins to suggest a framework for future work at any organization working on reducing delays and waiting times in these areas.

Obstacles and Solutions Reducing

	Obstacle 1 Cases Vary in Length and Predictability	Obstacle 2 Rooms, Not People, Are Seen as the Constraint	Obstacle 3 Processes Are Not Synchronized
SOLUTION A	Use control charts to study variation in case length.	Optimize surgery team utilization rather than operating room utilization.	Define start time for a case as the incision time.
SOLUTION B	Identify and eliminate special causes.	Do not equate an open room with a staffed room.	Define tasks and lead-times for each member of the surgical team relative to the incision time.
SOLUTION C	Estimate the capability of the process with respect to case length.	Standardize rooms to maximize their flexibility.	Remove barriers to adhering to the incision time and hold people accountable for compliance with the time.
SOLUTION D	Schedule unpredictable cases at the end of the day or in a separate room.	Reduce turnover time between cases by doing tasks in parallel and converting internal tasks to external.	Foster cooperation among professionals to help with contingencies.
SOLUTION E		Invest in "excess" equipment to support flexible use of surgical staff.	Standardize the preoperative process with the physician's office.
SOLUTION F		Stagger starting times for first cases of the day.	

Delays in Surgery

Obstacle 4 Late Cases Affect Subsequent Cases	Obstacle 5 Everyone Wants the Popular Times	Obstacle 6 Systems Are Not Coordinated
Have flexible movement of surgery teams among rooms.	Use data to illustrate the negative effect of uneven use of resources.	Design schedules to optimize satisfaction of the patient and the entire surgical team.
Study reasons for delays and focus improvement efforts on unnecessary delays.	Rotate unpopular times among physicians.	Standardize the preoperative testing and information process between the surgeon's office and the hospital.
Use one room for unavoidable contingencies.	Define cases that could be done beneficially at unpopular times.	Automate the transfer of information between the surgeon's office and the hospital.
Schedule unpredictable cases late in the day or in a designated room. (Tip: Do not emphasize efficiency in this room.)	Use pricing or other incentives to fill unpopular times.	Reduce variation in procedures and requirements at different hospitals in the community.
If subsequent cases will be delayed, alert hospital personnel, as well as patients and their families, as soon as the delay is known.		Make logistical information available at the surgeon's office.

Reducing Delays in Surgery

Obstacle 1

Cases Vary in Length and Predictability

Scheduling surgical cases and adhering to the schedule during the course of the day are complicated by the fact that the demand for surgery appointments is often unpredictable and the length of the surgery itself varies.

CHANGES TO OVERCOME THE OBSTACLE

SOLUTION 1A

Use control charts to study variation in case length.

Change Concepts:
Improve Predictions
Smooth the Work Flow

Organizations that have applied this improvement:
Beth Israel Deaconess Medical Center–West Campus
Dartmouth-Hitchcock Medical Center
Sewickley Valley Hospital

Control charts are used to plot data over time to identify the normal variation in a system (common cause variation), as well as variation that is due to unusual or unpredictable cases (special cause variation). In surgery, a control chart can be used to study variation in given types of cases, variation among surgeons, and other sources of variation.

The control chart analysis provides estimates of the variation that must be taken into account in scheduling and other processes. In addition, the analysis can lead to changes that reduce the variation.

SOLUTION 1B

Identify and eliminate special causes.

Change Concept:
Use Contingency Plans

Organizations that have applied this improvement:
Sewickley Valley Hospital

Special causes of variation in surgery may include the following: routine cases that develop unpredictable complications, unexpected shortages of staff, last-minute changes in physician schedules, and unavailable or malfunctioning equipment. These special causes of delay are not predictable, but they can be eliminated or minimized by building contingencies into the surgical system to reduce their impact on the system.

SOLUTION 1C

Estimate the capability of the process with respect to case length.

Change Concepts:
Improve Predictions
Identify and Manage the Constraint

Organizations that have applied this improvement:
Dartmouth-Hitchcock Medical Center

Tip: Begin with high-volume cases or particularly troublesome cases.

Scheduling too many cases by underestimating how long they will really take or by not allowing for variation in case length for potentially troublesome cases overtaxes the system, leading to delays. Estimate the capability of the surgical process to handle a given number of cases by taking into account the constraints (e.g., high-volume cases or those that are known to be particularly troublesome) at the start of the scheduling process.

SOLUTION 1D

Schedule unpredictable cases at the end of the day or in a separate room.

Change Concepts:
Use Multiple Processes
Identify and Manage the Constraint

Organizations that have applied this improvement:
Beth Israel Deaconess Medical Center–West Campus
Dartmouth-Hitchcock Medical Center
Sewickley Valley Hospital

Once a delay occurs during the course of the day, it is often difficult to make up the lost time. One way to handle cases that could have an adverse impact on the surgical timetable is to isolate them from the rest of the cases by scheduling them either at the end of the day or in a separate room. This minimizes their impact on the start of other cases.

Reducing Delays in Surgery

Obstacle 2

Rooms, Not People, Are Seen as the Constraint

In reducing surgical delays, people—the surgeon and surgical support staff—are the scarce resource. Often, however, because surgical suites involve heavy investments in capital equipment, the rooms and the equipment are mistakenly considered the constraint and are optimized at the expense of staff and surgeon time. This results in delays, with staff idle while waiting for available rooms. An alternative strategy is to maximize staff time, making sure that rooms are always available when needed.

CHANGES TO OVERCOME THE OBSTACLE

SOLUTION 2A

Optimize surgery team utilization rather than operating room utilization.

Change Concepts:
Smooth the Work Flow
Identify and Manage the Constraint

Organizations that have applied this improvement:
Beth Israel Deaconess Medical Center–West Campus
Sewickley Valley Hospital

One way to optimize the surgery team is to use flexible staffing of rooms, i.e., have more rooms available than staff at any given time so that, if necessary, staff can be moved into an open room. This makes the cases later in the day less sensitive to the cascading effect of a late case early in the day. In addition, flexible scheduling to accommodate same-day requests or requests for rescheduling by physicians, as well as flexible scheduling of OR support staff, can optimize the utilization of the surgery team rather than the operating rooms.

SOLUTION 2B

Do not equate an open room with a staffed room.

Change Concept:
Identify and Manage the Constraint

Organizations that have applied this improvement:
Beth Israel Deaconess Medical Center–West Campus
Columbia Wesley Medical Center
Sewickley Valley Hospital

The availability of a room for surgery involves the room being cleaned and stocked with the necessary equipment and supplies, and staff being available to support the surgery. This requires the synchronization of all tasks involved in the surgery process, including patient preparation. The availability of open rooms can be maximized by utilizing swing rooms that are not scheduled for cases but can be used when necessary.

SOLUTION 2C

Standardize rooms to maximize their flexibility.

Change Concept:
Use Multiple Processing Units

Operating room set-up time can be reduced by standardizing the equipment and supplies in all rooms, rather than requiring that the set-up be matched with each particular surgical case. Standardizing not only eliminates delays in room set-up, but also eliminates the need for designating particular rooms for certain types of surgery. (Such designation of rooms can lead to delays since it constrains the number of rooms available at any particular time.)

SOLUTION 2D

Reduce turnover time between cases by doing tasks in parallel and converting internal tasks to external.

Change Concepts:
Do Tasks in Parallel
Convert Internal Steps to External

Organizations that have applied this improvement:
Beth Israel Deaconess Medical Center - West Campus
Dartmouth-Hitchcock Medical Center
Sewickley Valley Hospital

Doing tasks in parallel (at the same time) rather than sequentially is an effective change concept for reducing delays in any system. In the surgical process, preparing rooms and patients in parallel can dramatically reduce delays in the preoperative process. This change may require the flexible use of surgical staff and the willingness of staff to see themselves as part of the same system and cooperate to achieve the desired results, e.g., the anesthesiologist inserting lines when support staff are busy.

SOLUTION 2E

Invest in "excess" equipment to support flexible use of surgical staff.

Change Concept:
Identify and Manage the Constraint

The ability to standardize room set-up requires the necessary equipment and supplies. If equipment and supplies are considered the scarce resource, then having the necessary equipment and supplies available when needed may be considered by some as "excess" equipment. However, if the surgical team is considered the scarce resource, then their ability to utilize the rooms and equipment becomes the main concern and the availability of necessary equipment is essential, rather than an "excess."

SOLUTION 2F

Stagger starting times for first cases of the day.

Change Concept:
Smooth the Work Flow

Organizations that have applied this improvement:
Sewickley Valley Hospital

The capacity of the surgical process can be matched to demand more effectively by smoothing the demand that occurs with the first cases of the day. In order to facilitate synchronization of all tasks, the first cases of the day are staggered. Rather than having all rooms start at 8:00 AM, some are scheduled to start at 7:45 AM, others at 8:15 AM.

Reducing Delays in Surgery

Obstacle 3

Processes Are Not Synchronized

Surgery, like any complex process, involves multiple subprocesses that are performed at different times and at differing speeds, resulting in a progression that is not smooth. Much time can be spent waiting for another subprocess to be completed. Each step of patient preparation for surgery is interdependent with all other steps. If one step is delayed, the entire surgery process will be delayed.

CHANGES TO OVERCOME THE OBSTACLE

SOLUTION 3A

Define start time for a case as the incision time.

Change Concept:
Synchronize

Organizations that have applied this improvement:
Beth Israel Deaconess Medical Center–West Campus
Sewickley Valley Hospital

A common reference point is needed to ensure that all the subprocesses of the surgery process, including patient registration, pre-anesthesia preparation, room set-up, anesthesia, the surgery itself, and post-anesthesia care, come together. A first important step is to reach agreement that start time of a case should be defined rather than simply listed as "to follow." A second step is to agree on what that definition should be. Definitions of start time currently in use include patient in room, induction time, and incision time. The incision time should be the definition of start time for two reasons: 1) all preparatory tasks must be completed at this time, and 2) after that time, synchronization is made easier because all providers are nearby.

SOLUTION 3B

Define tasks and lead-times for each member of the surgical team relative to the incision time.

Change Concept:
Synchronize

Organizations that have applied this improvement:
Sewickley Valley Hospital

Each member of the surgical team has clear tasks that are defined by their relationship with other related and intersecting tasks. The start time for a task is defined by subtracting the expected duration of the task from the incision time. For example, if incision time is scheduled to occur 90 minutes after arrival, then patient arrival has a lead-time of 90 minutes from incision; nurse assessment is complete at 60 minutes before incision; anesthesiologist assessment is complete at 45 minutes before incision; patient is brought to OR 30 minutes before incision; and incision occurs at "time zero."

SOLUTION 3C

Remove barriers to adhering to the incision time and hold people accountable for compliance with the time.

Change Concepts:
Synchronize
Consider People to Be in the Same System

Organizations that have applied this improvement:
Beth Israel Deaconess Medical Center–West Campus
Sewickley Valley Hospital

Comparing actual completion time to scheduled completion time for tasks in the surgical process in relation to the lead-time can help focus attention on those parts of the process that experience delays either consistently or intermittently. Potential problem areas include the escorting or transporting of patients from registration to outpatient surgery, preoperative assessment, anesthesiologist preparation, room set-up, availability of room following a previous case, or the surgeon's arriving late. A daily control chart plotting the difference between actual and scheduled start times for cases is also useful for gaining an overall perspective on the process. If the surgical team sees itself as part of the same system, it can discuss problems that arise, such as delays in patients being escorted from registration to the outpatient services area, and can implement solutions.

SOLUTION 3D

Foster cooperation among professionals to help with contingencies.

Change Concepts:
Consider People to Be in the Same System
Extend the Time of Specialists

Organizations that have applied this improvement:
Beth Israel Deaconess Medical Center–East Campus
Dartmouth-Hitchcock Medical Center
Sewickley Valley Hospital

The role of the anesthesiologist is often key to the smooth running of the surgical process. The willingness of anesthesiologists who are assigned to the operating room to help with preoperative assessment and preparation when necessary, or to give the patient report to the PACU instead of the nurse, are both examples of cooperation among professionals that can reduce delays. Another example is the use of all staff to assist with patient transport.

SOLUTION 3E

Standardize the preoperative process with the physician's office.

Change Concept:
Consider People to Be in the Same System

Organizations that have applied this improvement:
Beth Israel Deaconess Medical Center–East Campus
Beth Israel Deaconess Medical Center–West Campus
Sewickley Valley Hospital

Standardizing the preoperative assessment and testing with physicians' offices can result in reduced delays for patients either during their preoperative visit or on the day of surgery. Agreement on the testing that is necessary for certain patients and the process for obtaining the testing eliminates frustration and confusion for the patients, and eliminates the ordering of unnecessary tests.

Reducing Delays in Surgery

Obstacle 4

Late Cases Affect Subsequent Cases

If an operating room is fully booked for an entire day, then a delay of only a few minutes in each of several cases can have a ripple effect on the start of subsequent cases. In order to maximize the use of rooms and personnel, several steps can be taken to eliminate delays or minimize their impact.

CHANGES TO OVERCOME THE OBSTACLE

SOLUTION 4A

Have flexible movement of surgery teams among rooms.

Change Concepts:

Smooth the Work Flow

Identify and Manage the Constraint

Organizations that have applied this improvement:

Beth Israel Deaconess Medical Center–West Campus

Sewickley Valley Hospital

Assigning surgery teams (including physicians) only to certain rooms means that some rooms may be idle while waiting for staff, and staff may be idle while waiting for a room. This misalignment of resources has an impact on the timely start of subsequent cases. The movement of surgery teams to an available room when necessary smooths the process and reduces delays.

SOLUTION 4B

Study reasons for delays and focus improvement efforts on unnecessary delays.

Organizations that have applied this improvement:

Beth Israel Deaconess Medical Center–East Campus

Beth Israel Deaconess Medical Center–West Campus

Dartmouth-Hitchcock Medical Center

Sewickley Valley Hospital

A daily chart plotting the difference between actual and scheduled start times of cases provides an overall perspective on the process. Such a chart clearly identifies the points during the day when delays occurred and whether the scheduled start times for cases subsequent to a delay were restored. A team can do this analysis in conjunction with a review of the completion of scheduled subtasks to help identify and resolve specific problems.

SOLUTION 4C

Use one room for unavoidable contingencies.

Change Concepts:
Convert Internal Steps to External
Use Contingency Plans

Organizations that have applied this improvement:
Beth Israel Deaconess Medical Center–West Campus
Columbia Wesley Medical Center
Sewickley Valley Hospital
Wesley Medical Center

To minimize or eliminate the impact of one late case on subsequent cases, designate a room as available for the next case when a case takes longer than scheduled. This eliminates delaying the start of the next scheduled case until the previous case is completed.

SOLUTION 4D

Schedule unpredictable cases late in the day or in a designated room.

Change Concepts:
Use Contingency Plans
Smooth the Work Flow

Organizations that have applied this improvement:
Beth Israel Deaconess Medical Center–West Campus
Dartmouth-Hitchcock Medical Center
Sewickley Valley Hospital

Tip: Do not emphasize efficiency in this room.

The impact of delays associated with more complicated cases on the rest of the surgical schedule can be eliminated or minimized by scheduling these cases at the end of the day or in a room that is designated for these cases. While this designated room may not be used to its maximum capacity, its availability for contingencies is more important to the overall functioning of the system than is the efficient utilization of the designated room itself.

SOLUTION 4E

If subsequent cases will be delayed, alert hospital personnel, as well as patients and their families, as soon as the delay is known.

Change Concepts:
Smooth the Work Flow
Consider People to Be in the Same System

Organizations that have applied this improvement:
Dartmouth-Hitchcock Medical Center

While delays may not always be preventable, the impact that delays have on hospital staff as well as patients and their families can be minimized through timely communication. Surgery is a very stressful event; alerting patients and their families to the occurrence of a delay can help reduce the stress and improve the patient's and family's satisfaction with the surgical services. Notifying physicians and hospital staff can also help make adjustments for subsequent cases.

Reducing Delays in Surgery

Obstacle 5

Everyone Wants the Popular Times

Systems function more smoothly when the demand is spread out over a longer period of time. When the demand is concentrated during certain times, the system cannot be fully maximized. Physicians often compete for popular time slots for surgery, resulting in overbooking rooms and overtaxing support staff. There are several approaches to managing this situation.

CHANGES TO OVERCOME THE OBSTACLE

SOLUTION 5A

Use data to illustrate the negative effect of uneven use of resources.

Change Concept:
Consider People to Be in the Same System

Organizations that have applied this improvement:
Dartmouth-Hitchcock Medical Center

Sharing with physicians the control charts that show the difference between actual start times and scheduled start times can help illustrate the impact of delays. Of particular use are charts showing the difference in delays between times of the day or week that are overbooked and times when the schedule more accurately reflects the true capacity of the system.

SOLUTION 5B

Rotate unpopular times among physicians.

Change Concepts:
Consider People to Be in the Same System
Smooth the Work Flow

Organizations that have applied this improvement:
Sewickley Valley Hospital

One solution to the high demand for popular start times for surgery is a scheduling system that rotates different physicians into the most popular times slots on a regular basis. Physicians must see themselves as part of the system of surgical services and be willing to adjust their preferences in order to assure the optimization of the entire system.

SOLUTION 5C

Define cases that could be done beneficially at unpopular times.

Change Concept:

Consider People to Be in the Same System

Organizations that have applied this improvement:

Beth Israel Deaconess Medical Center–West Campus

Some specialists (such as podiatrists) who have extensive clinic responsibilities throughout the day may find it more convenient to schedule their surgeries later in the day so as not to interfere with their clinic appointments. In addition, a late afternoon surgery may minimize the delay for patients who are being transferred to an inpatient unit, since more inpatient beds are often available later in the day.

SOLUTION 5D

Use pricing or other incentives to fill unpopular times.

Change Concepts:

Consider People to Be in the Same System

Smooth the Work Flow

In addition to relying on physicians voluntarily adjusting their preferences for particular start times, incentives can be used to smooth out the demand on surgical scheduling. For example, physicians can be given preference for desired times or easier access to same-day scheduling if they are also willing to take less desirable times.

Reducing Delays in Surgery

Obstacle 6

Systems Are Not Coordinated

Surgery is a system that includes the surgeon, the patient, the hospital or surgical facility, and even the postsurgical rehabilitation facility. A smooth-running system requires coordination among all steps, for example, scheduling the surgery with the hospital and arranging for preadmission testing and other patient-related services.

CHANGES TO OVERCOME THE OBSTACLE

SOLUTION 6A

Design schedules to optimize satisfaction of the patient and the entire surgical team.

Change Concept:
Consider People to Be in the Same System

Recognizing that there are multiple customers of the surgical process (physicians, patients and their families, surgical support team, payers, employers, et al.) can lead to designing a surgical schedule that maximizes the needs and preferences of everyone involved. For example, some patients may prefer a late afternoon surgery for work-related or family-related reasons. The physician and hospital can work to arrange a schedule that best meets the patient's needs.

SOLUTION 6B

Standardize the preoperative testing and information process between the surgeon's office and the hospital.

Change Concept:
Use Multiple Processes

Organizations that have applied this improvement:
Dartmouth-Hitchcock Medical Center
Sewickley Valley Hospital

One way to streamline the preoperative testing process is to develop a standard preoperative assessment tool that distinguishes between patients who need to be seen preoperatively and those who may be seen by the anesthesiologist on the day of surgery.

SOLUTION 6C

Automate the transfer of information between the surgeon's office and the hospital.

Change Concept:
Use Automation

Organizations that have applied this improvement:
Dartmouth-Hitchcock Medical Center
Covenant Health Care System, Inc.

If patients are screened initially in the physician's office for the appropriate level of preoperative testing, this information can then be transmitted to the hospital's preadmission testing staff electronically. This reduces delays in transmitting paper records, allowing for more timely follow-up with patients, scheduling necessary preoperative testing, and scheduling services needed on the day of surgery.

SOLUTION 6D

Reduce variation in procedures and requirements at different hospitals in the community.

Change Concept:
Consider People to Be in the Same System

The surgical system in a community may include many hospitals and surgical facilities. Reducing the variation in the procedures and requirements (for example, the screening required for preadmission testing) across the different hospitals in a community reduces the work required from the physician's office and streamlines the transfer of information between physicians and hospitals.

SOLUTION 6E

Make logistical information available at the surgeon's office.

Change Concept:
Minimize Handoffs

Organizations that have applied this improvement:
Dartmouth-Hitchcock Medical Center

Patients need to know the procedures for preadmission testing and admission on the day of surgery. Having this information available at the physician's office meets the needs of the patient and reduces work for the physician's office staff, which would have to call the hospital to obtain the needed information for each patient.

Measures Reducing Delays in Surgery

STANDARD MEASURES

Figure 4.1
LEAD-TIME TO SCHEDULE ELECTIVE SURGERY

Sample Figure

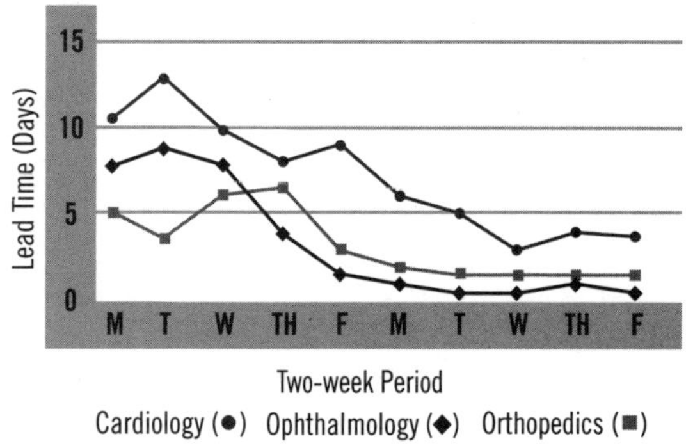

1. Lead-time to schedule an elective case

This is a measure of the number of days from the surgeon's call to the date for which the case is scheduled—in some cases a few days, in others up to a couple of weeks. A true measure of delay would be the difference between the surgeon's preferred date and the actual date.

Figure 4.2
PREPROCEDURE TESTING: WAITING TIME VS. PROCESS TIME

Beth Israel Deaconess Medical Center–East Campus
Boston, MA

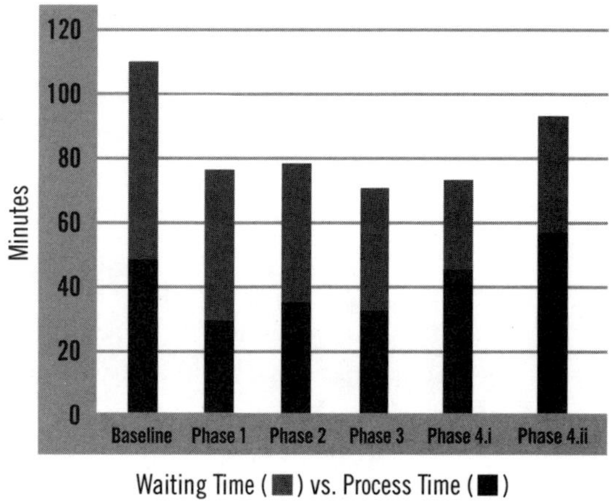

2. Length of separate preoperative visit

Factors contributing to long waits in preoperative testing include fixed order of the testing process, multiple types of preoperative testing, hard-to-sell time slots, limited provider availability, and variable process time. Figure 4.2 displays total time of preoperative testing, divided into process time (productive time) and waiting time.

Figure 4.3
CASE DISPLAY

Sample Figure
(Based on work at Sewickley Valley Hospital, Sewickley, PA)

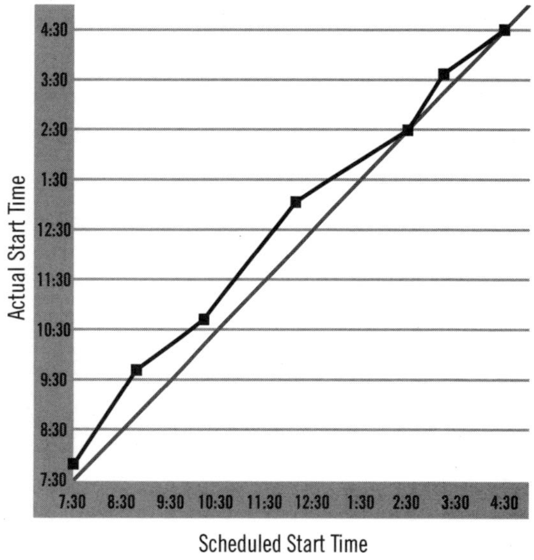

3. Delays on day of surgery: scheduled start time vs. actual start time

The Case Display graph is a simple way to display data comparing scheduled start time and actual start time for surgical cases. Cases above the 45 degree line are late; those below the line are ahead of schedule. The slope of the line between cases indicates whether the case took more or less time than scheduled.

BALANCING MEASURES

1. Percentage of patients needing a separate preoperative visit

In an attempt to streamline the process on the day of surgery, hospitals may push elements of the preoperative assessment check ordinarily done on the day of surgery to the preoperative visit prior to surgery. This may reduce delays on the day of surgery, but it might place a burden on the patient and cause more delays in the preoperative process by adding demand on that part of the system.

2. Percentage of cases cancelled on day of surgery

Cancellations on the day of surgery occur for a variety of reasons: unavailability of the surgeon due to other commitments, complications in the patient's condition, or incomplete preoperative assessment. Each of these is an indication of a breakdown in the system. Measuring cancellations over time is a way of checking on the overall functioning of the surgery process. Cancellations in the surgery log are tallied daily, including the operating room number and the reasons for cancellation. Data reflecting total cancellations can then be displayed in a run chart over several weeks or months, while reasons for cancellations can be displayed in bar charts or Pareto diagrams.

3. Cost per case

Cost per case is a function of the surgical staff paid by the organization, the cost of supplies and the cost of equipment. If staff are being underutilized, the cost per case will increase since productive time is being wasted. Cost per case is a balancing measure for reducing delays since it identifies systems that attempt to reduce delays simply by adding staff rather than by using staff more efficiently.

4. Provider satisfaction

Reducing surgical delays without regard to surgeon or other provider satisfaction may produce short-term solutions at the expense of the long-term success of the surgical service. Physicians function as both suppliers of services and customers of the hospital's surgical service. An ongoing measure of physician satisfaction will ensure that improvements in surgical processes are not made at the expense of physician satisfaction. Determinants of physician satisfaction include cases starting on time, ease of scheduling cases, ease of scheduling cases for the same day, working with the same support team, and the hospital's accommodation of the physician's preferences for day of week and time of day.

Obstacles and Solutions Reducing

	Obstacle 1 ED Has a Mix of Purposes	Obstacle 2 Demand for ED Services Varies	Obstacle 3 ED Provides a Variety of Services
SOLUTION A	Partner with a primary care group and refer patients to them.	Use historical data to estimate demand by month, day of week, and hour of day.	Focus on getting the patient to the exam room with the provider.
SOLUTION B	Have a primary care clinic on site.	Use estimates of demand to establish a staffing plan.	Establish multiple processes based on duration of exam and treatment.
SOLUTION C	Use ED waiting time to counsel the patient on other options for care in the future.	Establish contingency plans for unpredictable delays; call on staff from other parts of the hospital.	Study how physicians use their time and remove work that could be done by others.
SOLUTION D	Provide a process for an informative wait.	Be flexible in the use of house staff in teaching hospitals.	Establish protocols for top diagnoses.
SOLUTION E	Provide separate processes for short-duration treatment and observation of patients.		Based on protocols, initiate action at triage.
SOLUTION F			When the ED is not busy, have patients bypass triage and move directly to the exam room.

Delays in the Emergency Department

Obstacle 4 ED Is Dependent on Services Outside the ED	Obstacle 5 ED Is Dependent on Physicians Outside the ED	Obstacle 6 ED Is a Transition Point to Other Services
Move steps in the process closer together.	Establish and adhere to guidelines for response times to requests from the ED.	Designate the location of the next admit from the ED or inform the unit of the likelihood of an admission at the earliest possible time.
Assign x-ray technicians and/or phlebotomists to the ED.	Use protocols to anticipate the needs of the provider for tests or information to keep the process moving.	Develop and follow admission and discharge criteria for various levels of care.
Do simple chemical analyses in the ED.	Establish cooperation between the ED physician and the consultant to streamline the consulting process.	Fax the patient report from the ED whenever possible.
Assign leadership of an ED improvement team to someone from the supporting service.	If the patient is to be placed in an observation bed or admitted to the hospital, do the work-up or consultation at the destination point.	Move discharge times from the patient care units ahead of the busy admit times from the ED.
Match capacity of the supporting service to demand from the ED.		Assign a coordinator of patient placement.
Have staff observe "partner" departments.		

Reducing Delays in the ED

Obstacle 1

ED Has a Mix of Purposes

Emergency departments provide a wide range of services for people of different ages and backgrounds in the community, including trauma care, various types of urgent care, and primary care for some populations. Because the nature of the service varies constantly, it is difficult to streamline processes.

CHANGES TO OVERCOME THE OBSTACLE

SOLUTION 1A

Partner with a primary care group and refer patients to them.

Change Concepts:
Triage
Use Multiple Processes
Relocate the Demand

Organizations that have applied this improvement:
Chester County Hospital

For hospitals treating a large number of patients who use the emergency department for primary care, partnering with a primary care group practice or center may reduce inappropriate demand on the ED and provide a stable source of primary care for the patient.

SOLUTION 1B

Have a primary care clinic on site.

Change Concepts:
Triage
Relocate the Demand
Anticipate Demand

Having a primary care clinic on site eliminates the need for patients needing primary care to travel to another site, thereby eliminating the handoff of the patient from one site to another. Patients can often be seen immediately in the primary care clinic, possibly by midlevel providers using protocols, or can be given specific appointment times. Patients can be moved directly into primary care, rather than having to make an appointment and travel to a separate clinic location.

SOLUTION 1C

Use ED waiting time to counsel the patient on other options for care in the future.

Change Concepts:
Do Tasks in Parallel
Relocate the Demand

Organizations that have applied this improvement:
Kaiser Permanente

While patients are waiting for care in the ED, staff can provide them with information about urgent care centers, primary care centers, or group practices that could handle their needs in a more timely way than is possible in the ED. This time can also be used by hospital staff to gain information from the patients as to why they came to the ED for their care, such as proximity to their homes, lack of knowledge about alternative sites, or lack of a primary care provider.

SOLUTION 1D

Provide a process for an informative wait.

Change Concepts:
Automate
Do Tasks in Parallel
Promote Self-Care

Time spent in the ED waiting area can also be used for patient education on common conditions and preventive services, in addition to providing information on alternative treatment facilities. Videotapes, pamphlets, or other non-labor-intensive means of providing these services can be used.

SOLUTION 1E

Provide separate processes for short duration treatment and observation of patients.

Change Concept:
Use Multiple Processes

Organizations that have applied this improvement:
Beth Israel Deaconess Medical Center–East Campus
Chester County Hospital

Extensive waits for patients with urgent conditions that can be treated relatively quickly can be reduced by setting up separate processes for these patients. A Med Express or a fast-track system identifies these patients and moves them through triage and treatment as quickly as possible. Often a physician can treat a fast-track patient while waiting for test results for a more seriously ill or injured patient. A separate process can also be established for patients who require additional observation, such as patients with chest pain or asthma. Having an observation area or designated observation beds separates these patients from the rest of the ED and may also prevent unnecessary admissions.

Reducing Delays in the ED

Obstacle 2

Demand for ED Services Varies

Compared to the physician's office or clinic, the hospital emergency department has less control over when a patient comes in for treatment. In spite of this lack of control over demand, ED staff can take steps to match the capacity of their system to the varying nature of the demand by understanding whatever patterns of demand may exist and making adjustments in their system to handle the expected demand.

CHANGES TO OVERCOME THE OBSTACLE

SOLUTION 2A

Use historical data to estimate demand by month, day of week, and hour of day.

Change Concepts:
Adjust to Peak Demand
Improve Predictions

Organizations that have applied this improvement:
Chester County Hospital
Northwest Covenant Medical Center
St. Joseph's Mercy Hospitals and Health Services

Often, demand that appears to be completely unpredictable can be shown to have certain patterns once the data are analyzed. Plotting ED admissions by various time periods is useful in identifying whatever seasonal, weekly, or daily patterns may exist.

SOLUTION 2B

Use estimates of demand to establish a staffing plan.

Change Concepts:
Adjust to Peak Demand
Improve Predictions
Consider People to Be in the Same System

Organizations that have applied this improvement:
Chester County Hospital

Once the patterns of demand have been identified, the capacity of the system to handle the expected demand can be increased by arranging to have appropriate staff available during peak times. This includes not only direct ED staff but also ancillary services such as lab and radiology services.

SOLUTION 2C

Establish contingency plans for unpredictable delays; call on staff from other parts of the hospital.

Change Concepts:

Consider People to Be in the Same System

Adjust to Peak Demand

Use Contingency Plans

Balance Centralized and Decentralized Capacity

Organizations that have applied this improvement:

Columbia Wesley Medical Center

Even if patterns of peak demand can be identified and staffing patterns adjusted, there will undoubtedly be times when unexpected demand occurs. Having procedures in place whereby the ED can call on staff from other parts of the hospital to support them during unexpectedly high demand times can be an effective method for reducing delays. These procedures may also include admitting patients earlier than usual in the ED process, thereby relieving the back-up of patients waiting for treatment in the ED.

SOLUTION 2D

Be flexible in the use of house staff in teaching hospitals.

Change Concepts:

Extend the Time of Specialists

Use Multiple Processes

Organizations that have applied this improvement:

Cambridge Hospital

Academic medical centers have the challenge of providing patient care while at the same time training physicians. During high-demand times, the balance between these two missions often results in patient delays since it may take longer to coordinate care provided by a team of attendings and house staff. One solution during high-demand times is to have every third patient cared for directly by an attending physician rather than by the house staff. This, in effect, sets up a "physician express" system to move patients through the system quickly. In other situations, house staff can be called in to serve as an additional resource to supplement the ED staffing during times of particularly high demand. This approach is often used in clinic settings, but can also be applied to the ED.

Reducing Delays in the ED

Obstacle 3

ED Provides a Variety of Services

Emergency departments routinely provide a wide range of urgent care services, from stabilizing broken bones and closing lacerations to delivering emergency cardiac services and trauma care. Treating these patients requires synchronizing all the processes in the ED as well as in ancillary departments such as lab and radiology. Standardizing as many tasks as possible is an important part of achieving a synchronized care delivery system in the ED.

CHANGES TO OVERCOME THE OBSTACLE

SOLUTION 3A

Focus on getting the patient to the exam room with the provider.

Change Concept:
Synchronize

Organizations that have applied this improvement:
Children's Hospital, Boston
Columbia Wesley Medical Center
SSM/St. Mary's Health Center

Coming to agreement on the synchronization point, or the key reference point in any process, is crucial to achieving synchronization. In the ED, the point when the physician enters the exam room is the point around which everything else should revolve.

SOLUTION 3B

Establish multiple processes based on duration of exam and treatment.

Change Concepts:
Improve Predictions
Use Multiple Processes

Organizations that have applied this improvement:
Chester County Hospital
Christ Hospital
SSM/St. Mary's Health Center

An example of using a separate process for patients with similar exam and treatment times is the Med Express, or fast-track, system designed to expedite the movement of ED patients with urgent conditions requiring treatments of relatively short duration. The registration or triage nurse identifies these patients immediately upon admission and they are then evaluated and treated in a specially designed system aimed at minimizing delays.

SOLUTION 3C

Study how physicians use their time and remove work that could be done by others.

Change Concepts:
Extend the Time of Specialists
Identify and Manage the Constraint

Organizations that have applied this improvement:
Chester County Hospital

Because physicians are often the scarce resource in a system or process, patients are often waiting for them. This creates a bottleneck. One way to eliminate or minimize delays associated with this bottleneck is to reevaluate the work done by physicians to see if parts of their duties can be assumed by others.

SOLUTION 3D

Establish protocols for top diagnoses.

Change Concepts:
Use Multiple Processes
Minimize Handoffs

Organizations that have applied this improvement:
Children's Hospital, Boston
Columbia Wesley Medical Center
Glens Falls Hospital
Northwest Covenant Medical Center
St. Joseph's Mercy Hospitals and Health Services

Protocols are a set of agreed-upon steps that are taken in the diagnosis and treatment of particular types of patients. Identifying the top 10 patient diagnoses that are seen in the ED and developing protocols for the diagnosis and treatment of these patients can greatly reduce delays by streamlining the handoff of patients from one step in the treatment process to another. Protocols can also be an effective method for identifying steps in the treatment process that can be provided by other professionals, rather than by physicians.

SOLUTION 3E

Based on protocols, initiate action at triage.

Change Concepts:
Use Multiple Processes
Minimize Handoffs

Organizations that have applied this improvement:
Children's Hospital, Boston
Columbia Wesley Medical Center
Glens Falls Hospital
Northwest Covenant Medical Center
St. Joseph's Mercy Hospitals and Health Services

Once a protocol has been agreed upon, a patient who is admitted to the ED with a condition for which a protocol is in place can be moved immediately through the steps of the protocol, eliminating the delays that often occur in ordering appropriate tests. For example, a person with an extremity injury can be moved directly to x-ray rather than waiting to be seen by a physician.

SOLUTION 3F

When the ED is not busy, have patients bypass triage and move directly to the exam room.

Change Concepts:
Triage
Minimize Handoffs

Organizations that have applied this improvement:
Children's Hospital, Boston

Triage is used to assure that those in need of immediate care are seen first. The triage step is appropriate when the number of patients exceeds the capacity of physicians to treat them. However, at times when the demand is not high, the triage step can be bypassed, with the patient moving directly to examination by a physician or nurse.

Reducing Delays in the ED

Obstacle 4

ED Is Dependent on Services Outside the ED

The emergency department in a hospital is often thought of as a self-contained unit, while in reality it is part of the larger system involving emergency medical technicians or paramedics, hospital patient care units and other hospital departments, laboratory, radiology, and other support services, community physicians, consultants (physician specialists and other professional disciplines), as well as patients, their families, and the communities in which they live. While a smooth-functioning ED depends on the services that many others in the wider system of care provide to the ED, this can be difficult to achieve since others may not see themselves as part of this wider vision of the ED system.

CHANGES TO OVERCOME THE OBSTACLE

SOLUTION 4A

Move steps in the process closer together.

Change Concepts:

Move Steps Closer Together

Consider People to Be in the Same System

Organizations that have applied this improvement:

Columbia Wesley Medical Center

St. Joseph's Mercy Hospitals and Health Services

One way to reduce delays in obtaining services from supporting departments in the hospital is to provide those services directly in the ED. For example, some emergency departments have dedicated radiology services located directly in, or close to, the ED. This eliminates delays associated with transport to the radiology department, the availability of equipment, and staff who are busy providing services to outpatients as well as inpatients.

SOLUTION 4B

Assign x-ray technicians and/or phlebotomists to the ED.

Change Concepts:

Smooth the Work Flow

Consider People to Be in the Same System

Organizations that have applied this improvement:

Children's Hospital, Boston

Columbia Wesley Medical Center

St. Joseph's Mercy Hospitals and Health Services

This is an intermediate solution between having radiology and lab services actually located in the ED and having to call for an x-ray technician or phlebotomist to come to the ED when one is available. Having a technician assigned to the ED means that this technician's main responsibility is to respond to the demand for services from the ED, and the technician's secondary responsibility is to assist with other services for other patients.

SOLUTION 4C

Do simple chemical analyses in the ED.

Change Concepts:
Minimize Hand Offs
Move Steps Closer Together

Organizations that have applied this improvement:
Columbia Wesley Medical Center

Rather than sending all blood specimens to the lab for analysis, some EDs have the capability of doing some testing directly in the ED. This eliminates delays involved in having the blood drawn by a phlebotomist, transporting the specimen to the lab, and getting the results back from the lab.

SOLUTION 4D

Assign leadership of an ED improvement team to someone from the supporting service.

Change Concepts:
Consider People to Be in the Same System
Adjust to Peak Demand

Organizations that have applied this improvement:
Children's Hospital, Boston

Reducing delays in the ED is often defined as an "ED problem." If the improvement work is defined up front as an opportunity for other departments, such as lab, radiology, or patient care units, to improve their service to ED patients, then bottlenecks may be identified and eliminated more readily. For example, a patient care unit can study its high and low demand periods and shift its discharge times so that they do not overlap with a time for high admissions from the ED.

SOLUTION 4E

Match capacity of the supporting service to demand from the ED.

Change Concepts:
Adjust to Peak Demand
Consider People to Be in the Same System

Organizations that have applied this improvement:
Chester County Hospital
Children's Hospital, Boston
Christ Hospital
St. Joseph's Mercy Hospitals and Health Services
York Health System

In conjunction with the ED staff matching their staffing schedules to high-demand times, staff in supporting departments can realign their schedules and staffing patterns as well. One way to support efforts to align capacity and demand between the ED and supporting departments is to post ED patient waiting times in supporting departments. This gives supporting departments useful information and fosters the vision of everyone seeing themselves as being part of the same system.

SOLUTION 4F

Have staff observe "partner" departments.

Change Concept:
Consider People to Be in the Same System

As part of building an understanding of how the ED and other hospital departments and services are part of the same system, staff from one department can visit the related department to observe how the demand for services from one department affects the other. This can generate important information about how communication and patient handoffs can be streamlined and delays reduced.

Reducing Delays in the ED

Obstacle 5

ED Is Dependent on Physicians Outside the ED

Not only is the ED dependent on other hospital departments and support services, but it is also dependent on other physicians, particularly specialists, for interpreting lab and x-ray results and diagnosing and treating patients. Community physicians as well as specialists are often located outside of the ED, either in other parts of the hospital or even off-site. Developing clear lines of communication and protocols for initiating tests and treatments is essential for coordinating care of patients in the ED with both specialists and community physicians.

CHANGES TO OVERCOME THE OBSTACLE

SOLUTION 5A

Establish and adhere to guidelines for response times to requests from the ED.

Change Concepts:
Identify and Manage the Constraint
Consider People to Be in the Same System

Organizations that have applied this improvement:
Chester County Hospital

Usually physician specialists rotate responsibility for on-call duty for the ED. Delays often ensue when the designated on-call physician does not respond within the guidelines generated by the medical staff. ED staff, in conjunction with the medical staff, need clearly defined procedures for contacting an alternate physician if the on-call physician is not available for consultation.

SOLUTION 5B

Use protocols to anticipate the needs of the provider or specialist for tests or information to keep the process moving.

Change Concepts:
Minimize Handoffs
Smooth the Work Flow

When a cardiologist is called to consult on a patient who arrived in the emergency department with chest pain, the results of an EKG and other tests are essential for a diagnosis and treatment plan. Determining the needed tests at the outset can reduce unnecessary delays in getting the needed information to a consulting physician. Getting the results of tests to the physician immediately is an essential step in this process.

SOLUTION 5C

Establish cooperation between the ED physician and the consultant to streamline the consulting process.

Change Concepts:

Consider People to Be in the Same System

Extend the Time of Specialists

There is often variation across hospitals in the level of consultation needed before treatment can begin. For example, with chest pain patients, some cardiologists will order thrombolytics over the phone once they have received the test results from the ED physicians, while other cardiologists prefer to come in to the hospital to examine the patient and view the test results on-site. Consultants need to cooperate with ED physicians to facilitate the consulting process.

SOLUTION 5D

If the patient is to be placed in an observation bed or admitted to the hospital, do the work-up or consultation at the destination point.

Change Concept:

Convert Internal Steps to External

If it is clear that the patient needs to be admitted or should be moved to an observation bed, scarce resources in the ED can be freed by moving the patient immediately rather than waiting until all testing and consultations are completed. This requires coordination between the consulting or admitting physician and the ED physician, including agreement in advance about procedures for ordering necessary tests and requesting consults.

Reducing Delays in the ED

Obstacle 6

ED Is a Transition Point to Other Services

The Emergency Department is a transitional treatment site, with the disposition of the patient to another treatment location or to discharge being the end point in the ED process. Delays occur not only in diagnosis and treatment in the ED itself but also in moving the patient from the ED to another point of service in the hospital. Eliminating delays in sending the patient from the ED to the next point of service requires coordination, with each point of service seeing itself as part of the same system.

CHANGES TO OVERCOME THE OBSTACLE

SOLUTION 6A

Designate the location of the next admit from the ED or inform the unit of the likelihood of an admission at the earliest possible time.

Change Concepts:
Use Pull Systems
Consider People to Be in the Same System

Organizations that have applied this improvement:
Chester County Hospital
Christ Hospital
SSM/St. Mary's Hospital Health Center
York Health System

Staff of the unit that is the destination of the patient admitted from the emergency department experience the arriving patient as a new demand on its system. This demand can be handled more smoothly if that next unit can be given advance warning of the arriving patient. Staff at this location can then prepare their system for the arrival of the patient. Establishing a Be-a-Bed-Ahead system is the most efficient way to transition patients. With this system, the receiving unit anticipates demand and has an open bed available in advance of the request from the ED.

SOLUTION 6B

Develop and follow admission and discharge criteria for various levels of care.

Change Concepts:
Use Pull Systems
Consider People to Be in the Same System

Organizations that have applied this improvement:
Christ Hospital
York Health System

A potential barrier to moving patients from one point of care to another is the availability of beds in the receiving unit. In moving patients from the ED to the ICU and/or telemetry beds, hospitals have found that one way to ensure that a bed is available in these units is to establish and review regularly the discharge criteria for these units. Availability can be increased by adhering to the agreed-upon criteria, e.g., by not keeping patients in ICU or telemetry longer than is necessary.

SOLUTION 6C

Fax the patient report from the ED whenever possible.

Change Concept:
Use Automation

Organizations that have applied this improvement:
Beth Israel Deaconess Medical Center–East Campus
Children's Hospital, Boston

Delays often occur in transferring patients when the nurse on the receiving floor is not available to take the patient report from the ED. This problem can be eliminated by agreeing that all patient reports will be faxed to the receiving department, unless there is some special information that needs to be conveyed directly.

SOLUTION 6D

Move discharge times from the patient care units ahead of the busy admit times from the ED.

Change Concepts:
Improve Predictions
Consider People to Be in the Same System
Adjust to Peak Demand

Organizations that have applied this improvement:
Children's Hospital, Boston
Franciscan Skemp Healthcare–Mayo health System
SSM/St. Francis Hospital & Health Center
York Health System

Delays result when discharge times on inpatient care units do not precede busy ED admit times. Patients are queued and wait to be transferred to a department where patients are still occupying beds. Analyzing data on the peak admit and discharge times for the ED and patient floors can help to eliminate this problem.

SOLUTION 6E

Assign a coordinator of patient placement.

Change Concepts:
Minimize Handoffs
Move Steps Closer Together
Smooth the Work Flow

Organizations that have applied this improvement:
Children's Hospital, Boston
York Health System

A coordinator of patient placement triages competing demands for inpatient beds (e.g., ED admissions, postoperative patients, ICU transfers, elective admissions). In addition, this person assists in matching capacity to demand by coordinating staff and prioritizing patient flow through the system.

Measures Reducing Delays in the

STANDARD MEASURES

Figure 4.4
AVG. TRIAGE TO DISCHARGE FROM ED, ADMITTED PATIENTS VS. DISCHARGED PATIENTS

Children's Hospital
Boston, MA

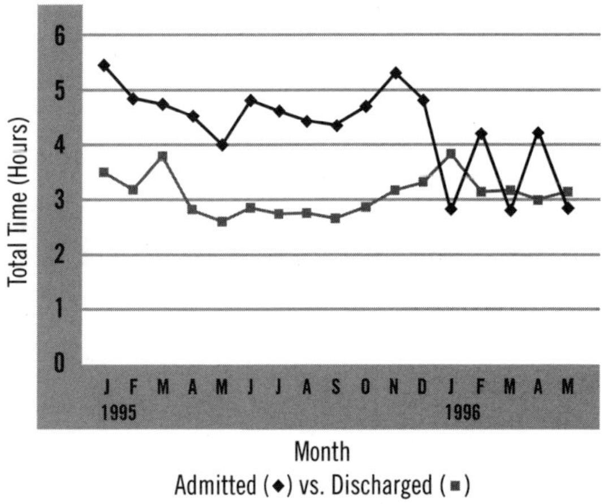

1. Duration of entire visit or part of the process

This measure includes waiting time and process time for all of the steps in the process (arrival, triage, registration, exam, consults and testing, clinical decision making, and disposition). Subprocesses such as "time from arrival to exam" may also be measured and tracked separately, in order to improve specific aspects of the process.

Figure 4.5
TOTAL EXTREMITY TURNAROUND TIME

St. Joseph's Mercy Hospitals and Health Services
Clinton Township, MI

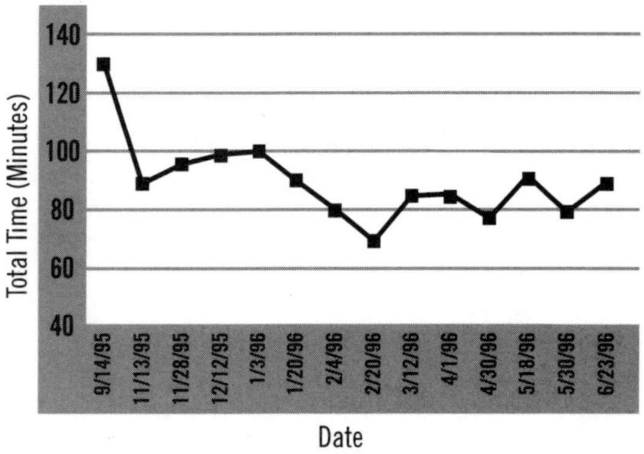

2. Duration of visit for particular problems

In addition to tracking duration of the visit for all patients, tracking the duration of the visit for a particular subgroup of patients—for example, patients with injuries to extremities—helps to identify delays that are associated with the treatment of a specific condition.

Figure 4.6
MEDIAN HOLDING TIME TO BE ADMITTED TO UNITS 6E, 6M, AND 7S

York Health System
York, PA

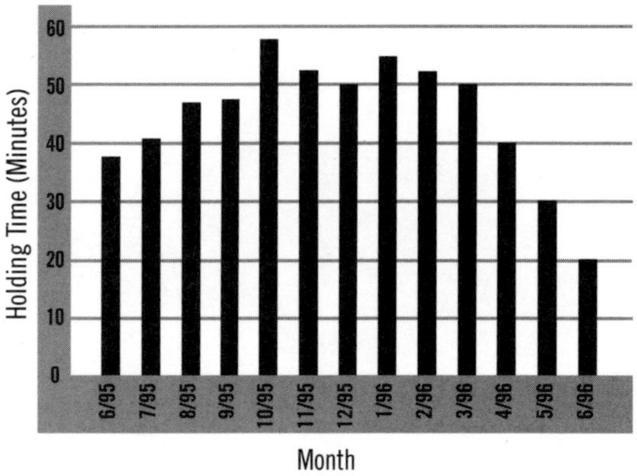

3. Duration of time from transfer or admit order to actual transfer to inpatient unit

This measure often reflects the effects of systems outside of the ED itself; patients may be delayed because inpatient beds are not yet available. Separating this measure from the overall delay in the ED can help teams work with the inpatient units to develop effective systems to move patients out of the ED.

Emergency Department

BALANCING MEASURES

1. Volume of patients

The volume of patients affects delays in the ED since an increase in demand without corresponding adjustments in capacity will result in delays. The effect of volume must be taken into account when measuring ED delays over time. Volume can be measured by charting the total number of ED admissions by hour of day or by shift.

2. Distribution of severity

The mix of patients seen in the ED also affects delays, since patients with more complex cases require more resources and staff time than do patients with less complex cases. Changes in this mix could be reflected in the measures of delays. If the hospital has an ED-based severity system built into its information services system, it can track the severity levels rather easily. Some nursing services use a system based on relative value units (RVUs) to measure the level of service intensity required for each patient visit. In the absence of a formal severity measurement system, diagnoses can serve as a crude measure of severity. For example, caring for patients with more severe conditions such as multiple fractures and cardiac arrest will consume more resources than caring for patients with relatively minor conditions such as simple fractures or lacerations.

3. Staffing ratios

Staffing ratios are a measure of the capacity of the system to respond to demand. Not only do variations in demand, as reflected in patient volume and severity, have to be taken into account in measuring demand, but also the number and mix of staff available to treat patients at any given time. Inadequate matching of the number and mix of staff with patient demand can result in delays in the ED. Physician, nurse, and technician assignments (both in the ED and on-call status) can be recorded for each shift. The availability of ED support services such as lab and x-ray should also be recorded.

4. Hospital daily census

Hospital daily census (number of inpatient beds occupied) can affect delays in the ED since, during high census periods, patients may be held in the ED while awaiting available beds. The effect of a high census is especially reflected in the measurement of the duration of time from disposition to departure from the ED. The daily bed census measured at intervals throughout the day is calculated routinely in hospitals each day. This information can be obtained easily and matched to waiting time from disposition to departure.

Obstacles and Solutions Reducing

	Obstacle 1 Schedules Are Overbooked to Meet Patient Demand	Obstacle 2 Processes Are Not Synchronized	Obstacle 3 Physicians Are Unavailable
SOLUTION A	Study demand for same-day or next-day appointments as well as preferences throughout the day.	Define appointment time as the point when the physician enters the exam room.	Use flexible rounds in the hospital to allow other physicians to round for those with clinic duty.
SOLUTION B	Schedule appointments to match demand for same-day or next-day appointments.	Synchronize timing of other tasks to the appointment time.	Include time in the schedule for telephone consults.
SOLUTION C	Redistribute elective seasonal appointments such as school and camp physicals.	Divide responsibility for timely patient flow and information flow and do the tasks in parallel.	Include physician telephone consultations in productivity measures.
SOLUTION D	Use alternative providers and alternative settings.	Rearrange administrative tasks as necessary to accommodate timely flow of patients to see the physician.	Use other members of the care team to take phone calls or to keep patient flow moving.
SOLUTION E	Develop guidelines for follow-up appointments for various situations.	Use short "huddles" at the beginning of the day to preview the schedule and make adjustments.	Study reasons for interruptions to physicians and eliminate interruptions that do not contribute to patient care.
SOLUTION F			Establish contingency plans for emergencies that require physicians to be out of the office.

Waiting Times in Clinics and Offices

Obstacle 4 Demand for Urgent Care Varies	Obstacle 5 Patients' Needs Vary	
Study historical data as well as patient demographics.	When making the appointment, prompt the patient to indicate the needs that must be met during the visit.	
Allocate capacity to serve predicted demand for same-day appointments.	Identify patients who take an unusually long time with a physician and schedule longer appointments for them.	
Designate a physician or a team to extend hours when demand exceeds capacity, and rotate this responsibility fairly.	Identify preventive or other services that can be performed if time permits after addressing the chief complaint.	
Establish flexibility among physicians and care teams to see each other's patients and give patients a choice.		
Adjust capacity to account for predictable seasonal fluctuations.		

Reducing Waiting Times in Clinics and Offices

Obstacle 1

Schedules Are Overbooked to Meet Patient Demand

Overbooking is often used as a method to meet access goals and accommodate patient requests for urgent appointments. However, overbooking causes patient delays in the office since it creates a greater demand than the system can handle. A number of methods for avoiding the need for overbooking involve shaping demand so that patients' requests for appointments can be accommodated within the normal scheduling system.

CHANGES TO OVERCOME THE OBSTACLE

SOLUTION 1A

Study demand for same-day or next-day appointments as well as preferences throughout the day.

Change Concepts:
Adjust to Peak Demand
Improve Predictions

Organizations that have applied this improvement:
Cambridge Hospital; GHMA Medical Centers/HealthPartners of Southern Arizona; Group Health Cooperative of Puget Sound; HealthPartners, Kaiser Permanente; MetroHealth; Virginia Mason Medical Center

Studying demand for appointments allows for a rough prediction of how many slots will be needed on any given day, or for a given week or month. The appropriate number of slots can be held open in anticipation of the expected demand so that patients' needs can be accommodated without overbooking.

SOLUTION 1B

Schedule appointments to match demand for same-day or next-day appointments.

Change Concepts:
Adjust to Peak Demand
Improve Predictions

Organizations that have applied this improvement:
GHMA Medical Centers/HealthPartners of Southern Arizona; Group Health Cooperative of Puget Sound; HealthPartners; Kaiser Permanente; MetroHealth

Keeping 30% to 50% of all slots open for same- or next-day appointments each day seems to be an appropriate range in primary care. The exact number of slots to keep open can be determined by each clinic or office practice by analyzing the patterns of patient demand for appointments.

SOLUTION 1C

Redistribute elective seasonal appointments such as school and camp physicals.

Change Concepts:
Smooth the Work Flow
Improve Predictions

Organizations that have applied this improvement:
Cambridge Hospital

Certain types of appointments, such as school and camp physicals, flu shots and travel-related immunizations, peak at certain times of the year. Anticipating this demand and soliciting appointments prior to the highest demand periods can help keep appointment slots open to handle more routine demand.

SOLUTION 1D

Use alternative providers and alternative settings.

Change Concepts:
Triage
Relocate the Demand
Promote Self-Care

Organizations that have applied this improvement:
GHMA Medical Centers/HealthPartners of Southern Arizona
Group Health Cooperative of Puget Sound
Kaiser Permanente
UNITYChoice Health Plan

Using alternative settings for care—for example, advice over the phone by a nurse or asthma education in schools—reduces demand on the system for appointments, once again allowing appointment slots to remain open for those needing to see a physician.

SOLUTION 1E

Develop guidelines for follow-up appointments for various situations.

Change Concept:
Extinguish Demand for Ineffective Care

Organizations that have applied this improvement:
Group Health Cooperative of Puget Sound
Kaiser Permanente
MetroHealth
University of Michigan Medical Center

To eliminate the routine ordering of follow-up or check-back appointments, develop guidelines that indicate when follow-up appointments are necessary and when a follow-up phone call might be sufficient. Patients can be given a date when they should call to see if a follow-up appointment is necessary. An appointment can then be made if the follow-up phone call indicates that the patient needs to be seen by the physician.

Reducing Waiting Times in Clinics and Offices

Obstacle 2

Processes Are Not Synchronized

As is the case with surgery and emergency department systems, the processes involved in a patient being seen in a clinic or office entail multiple stages that are done at different times and at differing paces. Many of the delays associated with office visits are related to the misalignment of the various steps in the process. Focusing all clinic or office processes on a single key reference point, i.e., when the patient is seen by the provider, can help bring the various steps in the process together, resulting in a more smoothly flowing system.

CHANGES TO OVERCOME THE OBSTACLE

SOLUTION 2A

Define appointment time as the point when the physician enters the exam room.

Change Concept:
Synchronize

Organizations that have applied this improvement:
Franciscan Skemp Healthcare–Mayo Health System
Virginia Mason Medical Center

Synchronization cannot occur unless there is agreement on the synchronization point, or reference point, for a system. Is the appointment time when the patient walks into the office? When he or she is seen by the nurse? When he or she is in the exam room waiting for the physician? Different people in the system have their own view of what the patient appointment time means. Agreeing that the key point in time is the point at which the physician enters the exam room is the first step in aligning all of the processes in the office or clinic.

SOLUTION 2B

Synchronize timing of other tasks to the appointment time.

Change Concept:
Synchronize

Organizations that have applied this improvement:
Franciscan Skemp Healthcare–Mayo Health System
HealthPartners
MetroHealth
Virginia Mason Medical Center

Tasks involved in an office visit that must be synchronized include the following: locating the patient's medical and financial records, bringing the medical record to the exam, preparing the exam room, documenting vital signs, and reviewing the reasons for the visit, and physician being available to see the patient. A patient experiences delays in waiting to see the physician when the start of a particular step in the process must wait for the completion of a previous step.

SOLUTION 2C

Divide responsibility for timely patient flow and information flow and do the tasks in parallel.

Change Concepts:

Use Multiple Processes

Do Tasks in Parallel

Organizations that have applied this improvement:

MultiHealth

University of Michigan Medical Center

Virginia Mason Medical Center

Because the tasks involved in a patient visit include the flow of information as well as the movement of the patient through the system, it is often helpful to divide the responsibility for each task. For example, having the receptionist responsible for greeting the patient as well as retrieving the patient's medical record from the medical record area may result in delays.

Difficulty in locating one patient record may mean that five patients are suddenly backed up in the waiting room waiting to check in. Having the receptionist greet and escort the patient to the exam room and a clerk retrieve the medical record is another way to divide the responsibility.

Note: This change does not require additional staff. For example, consider a system that has two receptionists handling two patients: before the change, each receptionist is responsible for moving one patient and the information for that patient; after the change, one receptionist moves two patients, and the other receptionist moves two sets of information.

SOLUTION 2D

Rearrange administrative tasks as necessary to accommodate timely flow of patients to see the physician.

Change Concepts:

Identify and Manage the Constraint

Use Automation

Extend the Time of Specialists

Organizations that have applied this improvement:

Covenant Healthcare System, Inc.

University of Michigan Medical Center

If the physician is available and waiting to see the patient, paperwork on the patient can be completed at other points in the visit. In this case, the physician is the scarce resource that should not be left idle waiting for the patient. Automated preregistration can also reduce dramatically or even eliminate the registration process.

SOLUTION 2E

Use short "huddles" at the beginning of the day to preview the schedule and make adjustments.

Change Concepts:

Improve Predictions

Use Contingency Plans

Organizations that have applied this improvement:

HealthPartners

University of Michigan Medical Center

Watson Clinic LLP

Clinic and office staff can meet briefly at the beginning of each day to preview the daily schedule and make any contingency plans in anticipation of the day's events.

Reducing Waiting Times in Clinics and Offices

Obstacle 3

Physicians Are Unavailable

Note: See also the changes to overcome the same obstacle presented in the section on Increasing Access to Care.

There are a number of reasons why a physician may not be available as planned, including hospital rounds, administrative duties, telephone consultations with patients, as well as unexpected personal and family emergencies. However, there are a number of ways to maximize a physician's ability to see patients, thereby aligning the capacity of the system to meet patient demand.

CHANGES TO OVERCOME THE OBSTACLE

SOLUTION 3A

Use flexible rounds in the hospital to allow other physicians to round for those with clinic duty.

Change Concepts:
Extend the Time of Specialists
Identify and Manage the Constraint

Organizations that have applied this improvement:
MetroHealth

Flexible rounds allow physicians to cover each other's hospital responsibilities during an assigned clinic time. In this way, each individual physician does not have to leave the clinic during assigned hours to conduct hospital rounds.

SOLUTION 3B

Include time in the schedule for telephone consults.

Change Concepts:
Extend the Time of Specialists
Identify and Manage the Constraint

Organizations that have applied this improvement:
Group Health Cooperative of Puget Sound
HealthPartners
Virginia Mason Medical Center

Squeezing telephone consultations into a busy clinic or office schedule is another form of overbooking, since the physician is really trying to take care of several patients at once. This can be alleviated by building telephone consulting time into the daily schedule.

SOLUTION 3C

Include physician telephone consultations in productivity measures.

Change Concepts:
Identify and Manage the Constraint
Extend the Time of Specialists

Organizations that have applied this improvement:
Group Health Cooperative of Puget Sound

Often the patient in the exam room is waiting for a physician who is on the phone consulting with another patient. These phone consults can be built into the physician's schedule for the day, but only if this will not interfere with reaching his or her targeted number of patients. Phone consultations are often an effective way for physicians to shape demand by assessing a patient's condition and preventing unnecessary office visits, and therefore should be included in the physician's patient contact time.

SOLUTION 3D

Use other members of the care team to take phone calls or to keep patient flow moving.

Change Concepts:
Identify and Manage the Constraint
Extend the Time of Specialists

To reduce the distractions to physicians, other members of the care team can take phone calls and help direct appropriate requests for phone consults with physicians. They can also help shield the physician from administrative calls which could be handled more effectively at a later time.

SOLUTION 3E

Study reasons for interruptions to physicians and eliminate interruptions that do not contribute to patient care.

Change Concepts:
Identify and Manage the Constraint
Extend the Time of Specialists

Organizations that have applied this improvement:
GHMA Medical Centers/HealthPartners of Southern Arizona
Group Health Cooperative of Puget Sound
HealthPartners
MetroHealth
University of Michigan Medical Center
Virginia Mason Medical Center

Observing the course of a normal clinic or office visit day for a small number of physicians can be an effective way to identify some of the common causes of distractions. Interruptions not related to patient care can then be reduced or eliminated.

SOLUTION 3F

Establish contingency plans for emergencies that require physicians to be out of the office.

Change Concepts:
Identify and Manage the Constraint
Use Contingency Plans

Organizations that have applied this improvement:
Kaiser Permanente

Contingency plans might include a "physician of the day" who remains in the clinic to see patients until all patients requesting a same-day appointment are seen, or having physicians on call who can fill in for the clinic assignments of other physicians who are unexpectedly unavailable.

Reducing Waiting Times in Clinics and Offices

Obstacle 4

Demand for Urgent Care Varies

The need for urgent care at a clinic or primary care office may seem, by definition, to be unpredictable. However, given a particular patient population, the demand for immediate or same-day appointments may be anticipated.

CHANGES TO OVERCOME THE OBSTACLE

SOLUTION 4A

Study historical data as well as patient demographics.

Studying historical information about visits and patient demographics can often identify patterns of demand that can be accommodated by the appointment scheduling system.

Change Concepts:
Adjust to Peak Demand
Improve Predictions

Organizations that have applied this improvement:
Cambridge Hospital; GHMA Medical Centers/HealthPartners of Southern Arizona; Group Health Cooperative of Puget Sound; HealthPartners; Kaiser Permanente; MetroHealth; Virginia Mason Medical Center; Watson Clinic LLP

SOLUTION 4B

Allocate capacity to serve predicted demand for same-day appointments.

Once the demand for emergency or urgent visits is estimated, the appropriate number of slots for same-day appointments can be held each day in anticipation of the demand.

Change Concepts:
Adjust to Peak Demand
Improve Predictions

Organizations that have applied this improvement:
Cambridge Hospital, GHMA Medical Centers/HealthPartners of Southern Arizona, Group Health Cooperative of Puget Sound, HealthPartners, Kaiser Permanente, MetroHealth, Virginia Mason Medical Center, Watson Clinic LLP

SOLUTION 4C

Designate a physician or a team to extend hours when demand exceeds capacity, and rotate this responsibility fairly.

Change Concepts:
Consider People to Be in the Same System
Adjust to Peak Demand
Identify and Manage the Constraint

Organizations that have applied this improvement:
Kaiser Permanente
University of Michigan Medical Center

In spite of efforts to predict same-day demand, occasions may arise when demand exceeds capacity. In this case, as an alternative to overbooking, the unit can extend the hours when patients can be seen. Having a designated physician who will remain in the office until all patients are seen—a "jeopardy physician," in the jargon of one organization—is one method of accomplishing this.

SOLUTION 4D

Establish flexibility among physicians and care teams to see each other's patients and give patients a choice.

Change Concepts:
Identify and Manage the Constraint
Consider People to Be in the Same System

Organizations that have applied this improvement:
University of Michigan Medical Center

Delays in access to appointments as well as delays on the day of a visit may result if patients are assigned only to particular physicians. If one physician is late arriving at the office, for example, start times for patients throughout the day will be affected. An alternative is to give patients the choice of seeing another provider rather than waiting for their scheduled physician.

SOLUTION 4E

Adjust capacity to account for predictable seasonal fluctuations.

Change Concepts:
Adjust to Peak Demand
Improve Predictions

Organizations that have applied this improvement:
Cambridge Hospital

Certain times of the year may be associated with an increase in emergency or urgent visits, for example, ice storms in the winter or the beginning of spring or fall sports. These seasonal fluctuations can also be taken into account in the allotment of same-day visit slots in the schedule.

Reducing Waiting Times in Clinics and Offices

Obstacle 5

Patients' Needs Vary

Just as physicians vary in their practice styles, patients also vary in their clinical needs as well as their personal preferences. Older patients may want a longer time with a physician, while younger patients may want a quicker appointment. Patients with more complex conditions may require longer appointments, while patients with more routine needs can be treated more quickly.

CHANGES TO OVERCOME THE OBSTACLE

SOLUTION 5A

When making the appointment, prompt the patient to indicate the needs that must be met during the visit.

Change Concept:
Anticipate Demand

Organizations that have applied this improvement:
Group Health Cooperative of Puget Sound
University of Michigan Medical Center

Identifying the extent of the patient's needs at the time of scheduling the appointment allows for adjustments in the scheduling. A decision tree questionnaire can be a useful tool for clerks to anticipate all of the patient's needs, e.g., procedures, before the appointment is made.

SOLUTION 5B

Identify patients who take an unusually long time with a physician and schedule longer appointments for them.

Change Concepts:
Anticipate the Demand
Smooth the Work Flow

Often, older patients or those with more complex conditions require longer visits. Clinics and physicians' offices should identify these patients and schedule longer appointments for them.

SOLUTION 5C

Identify preventive or other services that can be performed if time permits after addressing the chief complaint.

Change Concepts:
Extend the Time of Specialists
Combine Services

Organizations that have applied this improvement:
Kaiser Permanente

To reduce future demand, preventive services such as flu shots can be performed during a patient visit if time permits.

Measures Reducing Waiting Times

STANDARD MEASURES

Figure 4.7
ACTUAL SCHEDULED APPOINTMENT VS. PHYSICIAN ENTERING THE EXAM ROOM

Franciscan Skemp Healthcare–Mayo Health System
La Crosse, WI

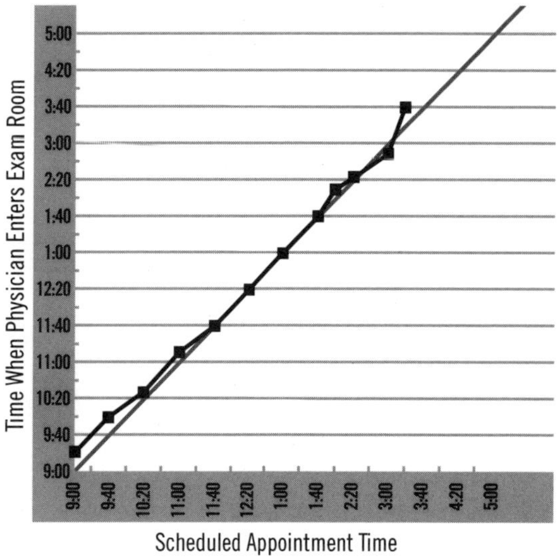

1. Scheduled appointment time vs. time physician enters the exam room

Comparing the scheduled appointment time with the time when the physician actually enters the exam room is a simple, effective way of answering the question, "Are we running on time?" Figure 4.7 shows at a glance when the physician is running late: that is when the line on the chart is above the 45 degree line. The slope of the line between cases indicates whether a patient took more or less time than scheduled.

Figure 4.8
WAITING TIME FROM APPOINTMENT TO PROVIDER IN ROOM

MetroHealth
Indianapolis, IN

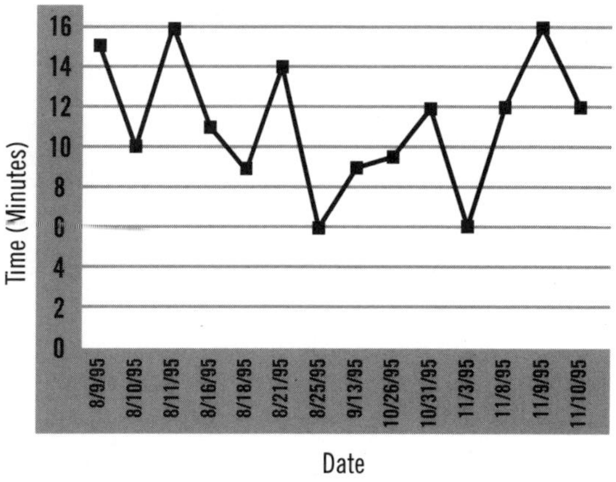

2. Delays in different parts of the process, for example, time to exam room

This graph measures steps in the process (patient arrives, patient brought to exam room, provider sees patient, provider transmits orders, orders completed, results delivered to provider, and next steps communicated to patient). The graph also identifies the longest delays and helps to focus improvement efforts on these areas.

Figure 4.9
PHONE DELAY: WAITING TIME TO ANSWER

Sample Figure

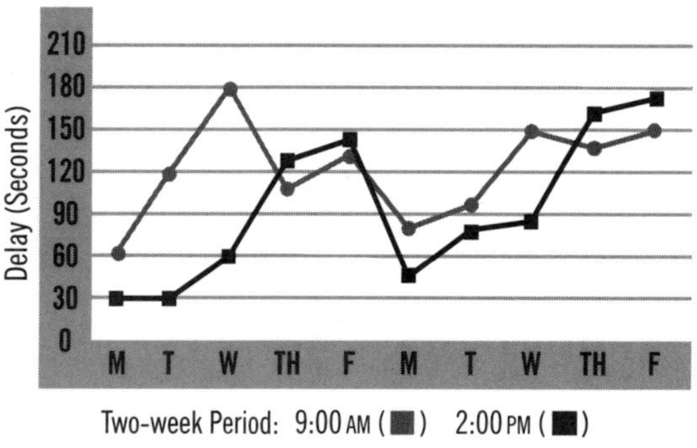

3. Phone delay

This measure tracks how long a patient waits on the phone to schedule an appointment or to get information from the office or clinic. A simple way to measure this is to pick two points during the day, make two calls each day for a week, and record the waiting time.

in Clinics and Physicians' Offices

BALANCING MEASURES

1. Lead-time by type of appointment

Measuring the time from when a patient requests an appointment until the time the appointment actually takes place provides a check on whether waiting time in clinics and offices is being shortened by decreasing access. Data for plotting lead-time can be collected either by the staff person who schedules appointments or by asking patients on the day of their appointment how long they waited for the appointment.

2. Over- or underutilization of appointment slots

Delays in accessing appointments can be reduced by overutilizing slots, i.e., by overbooking; this, however, contributes to delays on the day of the appointment. Underutilization of slots may result in less waiting time on the day of the appointment, but will result in greater costs for the clinic. Overutilization is measured by recording the number of double bookings per day. Measure underutilization by recording the number of appointment slots unused.

3. Patient satisfaction

Regular patient surveys monitor the effect of changes that are tested in reducing delays and waiting times. For example, if a clinic decides to reduce the waiting time in the reception area, but then doubles the amount of time the patient waits in the waiting room, this will be reflected in the patient survey of satisfaction with the overall waiting time.

4. Appointments cancelled by the clinic

Cancellations are a reflection of either a lack of provider capacity or a failure to balance the schedules of providers with scheduled appointments. The person who notifies patients of cancellations can keep a tally.

5. Cost

Waiting times in clinics and physicians' offices can be reduced using methods that increase costs, such as increasing the number of providers. If this is done instead of maximizing current capacity or shaping demand, then the result is unnecessary costs to the system.

6. Provider satisfaction

A survey of physicians, nurses, and other staff members can provide valuable information about the impact of changes made to reduce waiting times for patients. The needs of providers, particularly physicians, as customers of the clinics must be balanced with their role as suppliers of patient care.

Obstacles and Solutions Increasing

	Obstacle 1 Demand for Care Varies	Obstacle 2 Increasing Capacity Is Assumed to Be Costly	Obstacle 3 Physicians are Unavailable
SOLUTION A	Study demand for same-day or next-day appointments.	Identify and remove unnecessary interruptions and other inefficient uses of physicians' time.	Establish standards for hours per week and weeks per year in the clinic.
SOLUTION B	Use guidelines for demand in relation to panel size.	Offer specialty clinics, group appointments, or specified times for certain types of problems.	Obtain physicians' commitment to the schedule in advance and then restrict last-minute changes.
SOLUTION C	Use patient preferences as input for scheduling standard appointment times.	Redistribute elective seasonal appointments, such as school and camp physicals, to reduce surges in demand.	Curtail physicals and other elective appointments when physician capacity is low.
SOLUTION D	Allocate sufficient slots to provide for demand for same-day appointments.	Use alternative providers and alternative settings, for example, advice over the phone by a nurse.	
SOLUTION E	Match capacity of providers to predicted demand for services from various patient populations.	Assist people in self-care, for example, teaching asthma patients to adjust their medications based on peak flow meter results.	
SOLUTION F	Use measures of demand, appointment availability, overbooking, or overtime to adjust capacity.		

Access to Care

Obstacle 4 Physicians' Practice Styles Vary	Obstacle 5 Backlogs Clog the System	
Recognize and adapt to varying practice styles.	Use overtime or other extended hours to work down the backlog.	
Recognize that redesigning the system and shaping demand will usually have a bigger impact on productivity than focusing on individual practice styles.	Bring in other providers for a short period of time.	
Use productivity as one of a family of measures to evaluate the effectiveness of physicians.	Study the existing scheduled appointments and provide alternatives to office visits if appropriate.	
Use incentives based on a family of measures, including patient satisfaction.		
Use control charts to compare physicians' practices.		

Increasing Access to Care

Obstacle 1

Demand for Care Varies

Primary care and physician office practices have to respond to demand, particularly for same-day appointments, that often varies dramatically. While this demand may seem at first unpredictable, there are methods for understanding whatever patterns may exist and adjusting the clinic's capacity accordingly.

CHANGES TO OVERCOME THE OBSTACLE

SOLUTION 1A

Study demand for same-day or next-day appointments.

Some part of the demand for primary care appointments is unpredictable, but there may be patterns of demand that vary predictably by month, week, or day. Analyzing patients' calls requesting same-day appointments can help identify these patterns and help align provider availability with demand.

Change Concepts:
Adjust to Peak Demand
Improve Predictions

Organizations that have applied this improvement:
Cambridge Hospital; GHMA Medical Centers/HealthPartners of Southern Arizona; Group Health Cooperative of Puget Sound; HealthPartners; Kaiser Permanente; MetroHealth; Virginia Mason Medical Center; Watson Clinic LLP

SOLUTION 1B

Use guidelines for demand in relation to panel size.

Regression models and other methods or large databases are useful to predict demand. Guidelines can be used for matching provider capacity to demand based on the size and characteristics of a practice's patient base.

Change Concepts:
Adjust to Peak Demand
Improve Predictions

Organizations that have applied this improvement:
Group Health Cooperative of Puget Sound
Kaiser Permanente
Virginia Mason Medical Center

SOLUTION 1C

Use patient preferences as input for scheduling standard appointment times.

Change Concepts:
Improve Predictions
Use Multiple Processes

Keeping track of the time of day or the day of week that patients request appointments can be useful in developing a simple predictive model and offering these preferred times as standard appointment times. For example, if there is a high demand for evening appointments, a practice may consider offering several nights a week for evening appointments rather than just one.

SOLUTION 1D

Allocate sufficient slots to provide for demand for same-day appointments.

Change Concepts:
Smooth the Work Flow
Adjust to Peak Demand

Organizations that have applied this improvement:
GHMA Medical Centers/HealthPartners of Southern Arizona; Group Health Cooperative of Puget Sound; HealthPartners; Kaiser Permanente; MetroHealth

Once the range of the demand for same-day appointments is determined, including any seasonal variations, a clinic or office can block a sufficient number of appointment slots in anticipation of this demand. Allotting 30% to 50% of the appointment slots for a primary care office practice is an appropriate range.

SOLUTION 1E

Match capacity of providers to predicted demand for services from various patient populations.

Change Concepts:
Improve Predictions
Smooth the Work Flow

Organizations that have applied this improvement:
Cambridge Hospital; Department of Veterans Affairs Medical Center; GHMA Medical Centers/HealthPartners of Southern Arizona; Group Health Cooperative of Puget Sound; HealthPartners; Kaiser Permanente; MetroHealth; University of Michigan Medical Center; Virginia Mason Medical Center; Watson Clinic LLP

Knowing the demographic characteristics of your patient population can also help in predicting demand. For example, populations with a large percentage of patients age 20 to 40 might be expected to generate a greater demand for pediatric services than a population with a large concentration of elderly patients. Providers who are trained to meet the needs of specific patient populations can then be assigned a certain percentage of the appointment slots in anticipation of this demand.

SOLUTION 1F

Use measures of demand, appointment availability, overbooking, or overtime to adjust capacity.

Change Concepts:
Adjust to Peak Demand
Improve Predictions

Capacity, or the availability of providers, can be adjusted based on ongoing data collected from the office practice. Insufficient capacity often results in an increase in overbooking and an increase in overtime hours by physicians and office staff. Plotting these measures over time, with the help of control charts, is one method of continuously assessing the alignment of demand and capacity, and of guiding appropriate adjustments.

Increasing Access to Care

Obstacle 2

Increasing Capacity Is Assumed to Be Costly

Increasing capacity does not necessarily mean that additional resources, such as physicians or office staff, need to be added to the system. An alternative method for increasing capacity is to improve the efficiency of the current system.

CHANGES TO OVERCOME THE OBSTACLE

SOLUTION 2A

Identify and remove unnecessary interruptions and other inefficient uses of physicians' time.

Change Concepts:
Identify and Manage the Constraint
Extend the Time of Specialists

Organizations that have applied this improvement:
GHMA Medical Centers/HealthPartners of Southern Arizona
Group Health Cooperative of Puget Sound
HealthPartners
MetroHealth
Virginia Mason Medical Center

Physicians are usually the scarce resource in an office practice. Patients are ready in the waiting room, but the doctor is busy seeing other patients or taking care of other responsibilities, such as returning patients' phone calls. Physicians' time can be extended by identifying non-patient-care tasks performed by physicians during office hours, and either reassigning these tasks to other staff or arranging time outside of office hours for physicians to take care of administrative or hospital-related responsibilities.

SOLUTION 2B

Offer specialty clinics, group appointments, or specified times for certain types of problems.

Change Concepts:
Use Multiple Processes
Extend the Time of Specialists
Combine Services

Organizations that have applied this improvement:
Department of Veterans Affairs Medical Center
MetroHealth

Offering alternatives to individual appointments for patients with conditions that generate high demand for services—hypertension, for example is one approach to extending physicians' time and generating additional capacity in the system for the physician to see additional patients.

SOLUTION 2C

Redistribute elective seasonal appointments, such as school and camp physicals, to reduce surges in demand.

Change Concepts:
Adjust to Peak Demand
Improve Predictions
Smooth the Work Flow

Organizations that have applied this improvement:
Cambridge Hospital

Smoothing demand by spreading predictable appointments over longer periods of time can help increase the capacity of the system. Scheduling high school sports physicals throughout the summer instead of waiting until mid-August is one example of smoothing demand.

SOLUTION 2D

Use alternative providers and alternative settings, for example, advice over the phone by a nurse.

Change Concepts:
Automate
Triage

Organizations that have applied this improvement:
GHMA Medical Centers/HealthPartners of Southern Arizona
Group Health Cooperative of Puget Sound
HealthSystem Minnesota
Kaiser Permanente

Substituting the demand for an appointment by offering advice from a nurse or patient educational hotline is another approach to extending the capacity of the system while minimizing demand on its scarce resources, e.g., the physician and the individual appointment.

SOLUTION 2E

Assist people in self-care, for example, teaching asthma patients to adjust their medications based on peak flow meter results.

Change Concepts:
Promote Self-Care

Organizations that have applied this improvement:
GHMA Medical Centers/ HealthPartners of Southern Arizona
HealthSystem Minnesota
Kaiser Permanente
UNITYChoice Health Plan

Increasing patients' education and involvement in their own care, together with access to other levels of clinical advice such as nurse consultations, can reduce the demand on physician- and office-based services.

Increasing Access to Care

Obstacle 3

Physicians Are Unavailable

Note: See also the changes to overcome the same obstacle presented in the section on Reducing Waiting Times in Clinics and Physicians' Offices.

Many factors contribute to the unavailability of physicians for appointments. Physicians' hours in the primary care setting must be balanced with other demands on their time, including hospital rounds, teaching responsibilities, administrative duties as well as personal and family responsibilities. However, there are a number of steps that can be taken to maximize physicians' ability to see patients, thereby aligning the capacity of the system to meet patient demand.

CHANGES TO OVERCOME THE OBSTACLE

SOLUTION 3A

Establish standards for hours per week and weeks per year in the clinic.

Change Concepts:
Adjust to Peak Demand
Improve Predictions
Identify and Manage the Constraint

Organizations that have applied this improvement:
Deborah Heart & Lung Center
Group Health Cooperative of Puget Sound
Kaiser Permanente
Virginia Mason Medical Center

Once the size and patient characteristics of the clinic practice have been used to predict demand, it is possible to allocate the needed patient appointment slots in terms of number, time of day, and day of week. The number and type of physicians can then be matched with the scheduled appointment slots. Physician availability can be maximized by insuring that all physicians share responsibility for covering appointments in the clinic by establishing agreement among the medical staff as to the standard hours per week and weeks per year that they will be available to see patients.

SOLUTION 3B

Obtain physicians' commitment to the schedule in advance and then restrict last-minute changes.

Change Concepts:
Adjust to Peak Demand
Identify and Manage the Constraint

Organizations that have applied this improvement:
Cambridge Hospital
Kaiser Permanente
Virginia Mason Medical Center

Unexpected unavailability of physicians to staff the clinic can affect both a patient's ability to obtain a same-day appointment and the extent of delays on the day of the appointment itself. Restricting last-minute changes in physicians' schedules may be difficult, but the improvement in patient access and reduction of delays can be significant.

SOLUTION 3C

Curtail physicals and other elective appointments when physician capacity is low.

Change Concepts:
Adjust to Peak Demand
Extend the Time of Specialists
Identify and Manage the Constraint

When the full complement of physicians is not available, patient access to same-day appointments can still be maintained by limiting less urgent appointments, such as routine physicals, and scheduling these less urgent appointments for another time.

Increasing Access to Care

Obstacle 4

Physicians' Practice Styles Vary

One approach to increasing patient access to primary care is to establish a small number of possible appointment types with a corresponding time period for each, e.g., 15- or 30-minute appointments. However, the ability to set daily clinic schedules in this way is complicated by the fact that physician practice styles vary. One physician might take 30 minutes for a physical, while another might take 45 minutes.

CHANGES TO OVERCOME THE OBSTACLE

SOLUTION 4A

Recognize and adapt to varying practice styles.

Change Concept:
Match Capacity to Demand

Organizations that have applied this improvement:
HealthPartners
MetroHealth
Watson Clinic LLP

Physicians vary in the amount of time that they spend with patients, the amount of personal phone contact they have with patients, and the use of check-back appointments. This variation, if recognized, can be built into a scheduling system that accurately reflects how long a patient needs to be scheduled for an examination with a particular provider or how much time a physician needs to allow in his or her day to consult with patients. Similarly, patients vary in the amount of time they prefer to spend with physicians; clinics can stratify patients according to their needs and send patients to physicians whose style best suits the need.

SOLUTION 4B

Recognize that redesigning the system and shaping demand will usually have a bigger impact on productivity than focusing on individual practice styles.

Change Concepts:
Smooth the Work Flow
Extend the Time of Specialists
Identify and Manage the Constraint
Relocate the Demand

In addition to standardizing physician practices, there are several other methods for smoothing patient flow through the office. Changes such as relocating the demand for patients who can be given telephone consultations instead of coming in for an appointment, or anticipating seasonal demands by scheduling patients during slower periods of the year, can sometimes have a greater impact on productivity than changing the practice styles of individual physicians.

SOLUTION 4C

Use productivity as one of a family of measures to evaluate the effectiveness of physicians.

Change Concept:
Consider People to Be in the Same System

The number of patients a physician sees per day, week, month, and year, as a reflection of his or her productivity, is only one measure of a physician's effectiveness in providing care to patients. Other measures, such as patient satisfaction, the use of effective telephone care, how often a patient needs to return for follow-up visits, and the ability of chronic patients to function normally, are all examples of important elements of a physician's total contribution to the clinic or office practice.

SOLUTION 4D

Use incentives based on a family of measures, including patient satisfaction.

Change Concept:
Consider People to Be in the Same System

Organizations that have applied this improvement:
Kaiser Permanente

Physician compensation is increasingly being tied to performance. Evaluating the effectiveness of physicians can be done most appropriately by considering not only productivity (in terms of face-to-face encounters), but also patient satisfaction and other measures of quality of care, such as patient functional status.

SOLUTION 4E

Use control charts to compare physicians' practices.

Change Concept:
Identify and Manage the Constraint

Providing data to physicians that allow them to compare their treatment patterns or productivity measures with those of other physicians has been shown to be an effective method of influencing behavior. Control charts can be used to highlight such physician-specific data.

Increasing Access to Care

Obstacle 5

Backlogs Clog the System

Although an organization may redesign the system and match capacity to demand, as long as a backlog exists—a legacy from the old system—it will prevent the new system from getting improved results. Working down the backlog often requires increasing the capacity of the system temporarily in order to clear it of its residual demand, so that the new system can start with a clean slate.

CHANGES TO OVERCOME THE OBSTACLE

SOLUTION 5A

Use overtime or other extended hours to work down the backlog.

Change Concepts:
Smooth the Work Flow
Work Down the Backlog

Organizations that have applied this improvement:
Kaiser Permanente
University of Michigan Medical Center
Virginia Mason Medical Center

When patients call for same-day or routine appointments to a clinic whose appointments slots are fully booked, access is limited. One method to reduce the waiting time for access to appointments (without causing waiting room delays by double-booking) is to extend the hours that the clinic or office is open. This is done only for a limited time during which appointment slots for the coming weeks are held open to absorb the anticipated demand for future patient requests.

SOLUTION 5B

Bring in other providers for a short period of time.

Change Concepts:
Extend the Time of Specialists
Work Down the Backlog

Another method of working down the backlog of appointments is to bring in additional providers temporarily to help alleviate the demand.

SOLUTION 5C

Study the existing scheduled appointments and provide alternatives to office visits if appropriate.

Change Concepts:
Extinguish Demand for Ineffective Care
Work Down the Backlog

Organizations that have applied this improvement:
Group Health Cooperative of Puget Sound
Kaiser Permanente
MetroHealth

Appointment slots may be opened by assessing the reason for an already scheduled visit and determining if the patient's needs can be met in alternative ways. For example, if a patient has a checkback appointment, a follow-up phone call from a nurse to assess the patient's condition may help the physician determine whether or not the checkback appointment is necessary.

TO DETERMINE THE NUMBER OF DAYS TO WORK DOWN A BACKLOG USING THE TABLE BELOW:

1. Determine the backlog in days.

2. Determine the proportional increase in capacity.

- Proportional increase in capacity = (New service rate – Current service rate) / Current service rate
- The service rate is the average number of people seen per day.

Example:
Proportional increase in capacity = (75 people per day – 50 people per day) / 50 people per day = .5

Note: It is assumed that the current service rate matches the demand. If the demand changes when the backlog is being worked down, take this into account when determining the proportional increase in capacity. For example: the current services rate is 50 people per day. If the demand increases to 55, then the proportional increase in capacity would be calculated: (75 – 55) / 50 = .4

3. Locate the backlog in days and the proportional increase in capacity in the table.

Example:
Backlog in days = 20
Proportional increase in capacity = .5
Therefore, days to work down the backlog = 40

	Proportional Increase in Capacity							
Backlog (days)	.1	.2	.3	.4	.5	.6	.75	1
5	50	25	17	13	10	9	7	5
10	100	50	34	25	20	17	14	10
15	150	75	50	38	30	25	20	15
20	200	100	67	50	40	34	27	20
25	250	125	84	63	50	42	34	25
30	300	150	100	75	60	50	40	30
40	400	200	134	100	80	67	54	40
50	500	250	167	125	100	84	67	50
60	600	300	200	150	120	100	80	60
70	700	350	234	175	140	117	94	70
80	800	400	267	200	160	134	107	80
90	900	450	300	225	180	150	120	90
100	1000	500	334	250	200	167	134	100

Figure 4.10
DAYS TO WORK DOWN A BACKLOG

Sample Figure

Measures Increasing Access to Care

STANDARD MEASURES

Figure 4.11
LEAD-TIME FOR URGENT APPOINTMENTS BY CLINIC LOCATION

Sample Figure

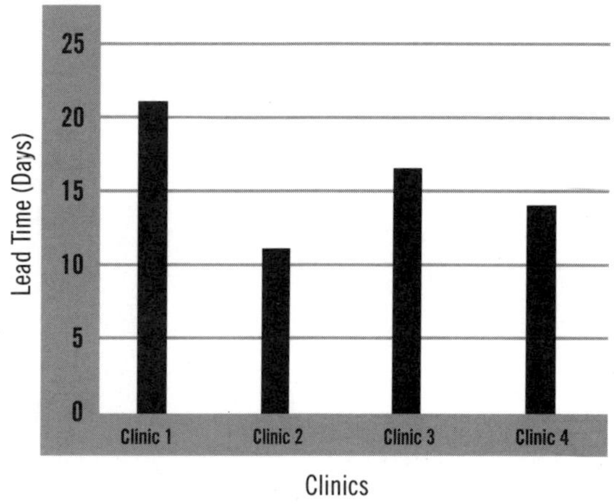

1. Lead-time

Lead-time is a measure of the time from when a patient requests an appointment until the time the appointment actually takes place. Optimal lead-time differs for different types of appointments. For example, an office practice may set as its aim meeting all requests for urgent appointments on the same day, while routine appointments are made within seven days of the time of the request.

Figure 4.12
LAG-TIME TO GET PHONE ADVICE

Sample Figure

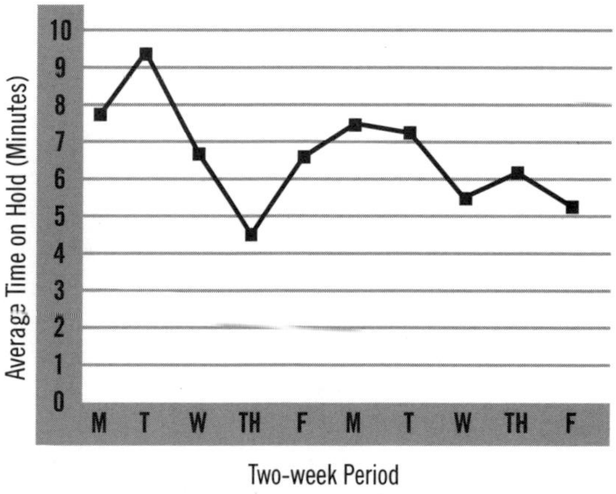

2. Lag-time to get phone advice

In order to shape demand effectively, office practices may establish a system to triage patient phone calls. Patients requesting an appointment are given one, while those needing advice about whether an appointment is necessary or about the appropriate site for treatment speak with a nurse. Lag-time measures the delays patients experience in getting the appropriate consultation.

Figure 4.13
OVERFLOW TO WALK-IN CLINIC AND ED

Sample Figure

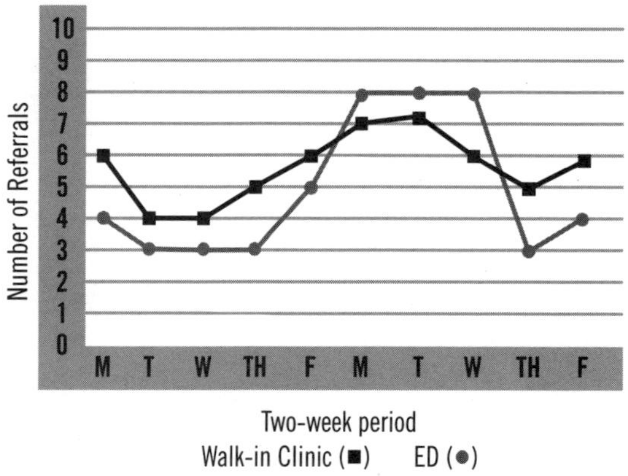

3. Overflow to walk-in clinic, ED, or after hours care

Record and plot the number of patients turned away from the primary care office or clinic because there were no open appointments. Plot this by day of week and by time of day. The receptionist could keep a log recording the time of the call and to which type of alternative site the patient was referred.

BALANCING MEASURES

1. Utilization of appointment slots

If appointment slots are being over-utilized, then patients will experience delays in obtaining an appointment. If appointment slots are being under-utilized, then there is more capacity in the system than is needed. Delays will not occur, but unnecessary resources are being used. In either case, demand is misaligned with capacity.

2. Delays in the clinic or office

One way to increase access is to make appointments for patients, even when there are no available slots; however, this will result in delays in the clinic. The goal is to increase access while reducing delays in the clinic or office.

Measure process time by having the patient or the provider record the time-in and time-out of each encounter with a provider. Waiting time can then be calculated as the difference between the process time and the total time of the visit.

3. Patient satisfaction

Patient satisfaction is a reflection of the methods used to increase access. For example, double booking results in increased access but may cause increased delays; patient satisfaction measures should reflect this.

4. Appointments cancelled by clinic

Access can be increased on paper by making appointments, but if the appointments have to be cancelled because providers are not available, access has not truly been increased. Once again, cancellations by the clinic are a reflection of a misalignment of capacity and demand.

5. Cost

Access can be increased using methods that increase costs, such as adding providers. If this is done instead of maximizing current capacity or shaping demand, then the result is unnecessary costs to the system.

6. Provider satisfaction

Efforts to increase access must be balanced with the needs of providers. Increasing access by double booking, for example, may get the patient an appointment, but will result in a frustrated medical staff, overscheduled with patients. Working with physicians to make realistic schedules that meet the needs of the patient as well as the medical and nursing staff will result in greater satisfaction of providers as well as patients.

All organizations attempting to change encounter barriers along the way, some large and some small. This section lists the problems that come up most frequently and solutions that have proven most effective.

Part 5

Troubleshooting: Overcoming Barriers to Change

Troubleshooting Overcoming Barriers

The commitment of senior leadership is probably the single most important variable in an organization's ability to achieve breakthrough improvement. Senior leadership commitment doesn't have to be time-consuming in order to be strong and effective. Here are nine simple but significant things senior leaders can do to create and sustain a culture of improvement.

HOW SENIOR LEADERS CAN HELP

1. **Establish "stretch aims" or "stretch goals."** Show by your constancy and your commitment that you intend to do what is necessary in the organization to achieve the new level of performance. State and restate the aims.

2. **Monitor the process frequently.** If you really want improvement to move fast, review progress daily, or hourly if necessary.

3. **Stay in touch with the improvement effort.** Support the team leader. Phone the leader. Pay specific, personal attention.

4. **Visit the team.** Drop in on meetings, even if only for a couple of minutes.

5. **Visit the site of the change.** Walk through the ICU or the clinic or the OR; show that you're aware of the improvement work being done. Look at the charts that are monitoring progress. Ask how you as an executive can be more helpful.

6. **Move the improvement effort up on the agenda.** Make it clear that improvement has high priority in the organization. A CEO who had been formally reviewing the progress of an improvement effort as #9 or #10 on the agenda moved it to #2. That simple act was a key factor in giving the project momentum.

7. **Assure that the team has the resources it needs.** For example, the team may need designated staff time or access to key data that others have collected.

8. **Celebrate successes.** Public celebrations of improvement efforts or personal expressions of appreciation are just as important as any modification of pay structure.

9. **Keep the bigger system in view.** The many local improvements are connected in a larger way to the system as a whole: it is the job of senior leaders to keep sight of, and help others to see, this larger context.

to Change

The problems (Dx, on the left) and solutions (Rx, on the right) are grouped according to the steps an organization must go through to reduce delays and waiting times.

Setting Aims

Dx	Rx
Aim is not a stretch.	Enlist the senior leader's help. The leader has the authority to take the status quo off the table and encourage the staff to move beyond "safe" goals.
Aim gets diluted over time; numerical targets are downgraded.	Resist the temptation to weaken goals. Identify barriers to progress and seek solutions instead of redefining the aim.
Initial aim statement is unclear, doesn't point to what action is necessary; no numerical targets are set.	Set numerical targets, and outline an approach and timeline for achieving them. If you can't see clearly how to plan changes or how to measure progress toward the aim, try redrafting it to make it more actionable.
Aims are multiple or lack unity.	Clarify aims. As long as the aims aren't conflicting, agree that the team will have a dual focus; work toward unifying aims as the project develops. If conflicting aims exist, enlist the aid of the senior leader.
Aim becomes unclear as work progresses.	Constantly focus on aims by repeating or reviewing aims at the beginning of each meeting.
Aim relates only to part of a system of care, but is not connected to the overall system.	Starting with parts of a system is okay, but be ready to expand the scope of the project once initial aims are achieved.

Establishing Measures

Dx	Rx
Lack of clarity about how to define and measure the primary outcome measure (e.g., delay in start of surgery cases, waiting time in physician's office).	Use the aim as a reference for defining the outcome measure. Aims should specify clear goals that reflect the change in the system. One approach is to define what you would like the results to show at the end of the project, and derive appropriate measures.
Confusion about the difference between outcome measures and process measures.	Use outcome measures, which tell whether the changes being made are leading to improvement, that is, helping to achieve the aim (e.g., holding time in ED).
	Use process measures, which tell whether a specific process change is having the intended effect (e.g., percentage of telemetry patients not meeting criteria for telemetry utilization).
Too many measures.	Make sure that measures match aims; evaluate whether you really need each measure to help guide changes.
	Collect only enough data to support the "study" phase of PDSA cycles.
Delays due to waiting for the information services department to provide data.	Use sampling instead of waiting for information services to crunch numbers. You can compare the results from sampling with those for all patients at a later time.
Limited access or no access to information services or to a computer system.	Use the resources available to you. Updating the organization's computer system is not a feasible endeavor for a short-term project; a great deal of change and improvement can occur using available resources and just enough data.
Lack of general interest in the data you're collecting.	Check on the clarity of and commitment to the aim.
	Present data simply (use graphs rather than tables).
	Don't collect too much data.
	Check whether the data help with PDSA cycles; if not, you're probably collecting the wrong data.

Dx	Rx
Resistance on the part of the staff to help collect or analyze data.	Make sure everyone has bought into the aims of the project.
	Make sure staff understand that data will be used for learning and improvement, not for judgment.
	Revisit the aims of the project and plan for testing changes; check whether you're collecting too much data, unnecessary data, or both.
	Make it easy for staff to collect data by integrating it into their daily routine.
Spending a majority of your time and energy on data (either collecting it or discussing it at meetings).	Emphasize using data in a test, with the focus on how data can guide the next PDSA cycle.
	Force an answer to the question, "What action could these data lead to?"
	Mandate a minimum data set and stick with it for a month.
	Use only available data.
	Suggest trying a PDSA cycle using existing data.
Resistance to small-scale data collection on the grounds of lack of "scientific" validity.	Differentiate between the level of data sophistication needed for research and that needed for improvement: randomized clinical trials are needed to establish standards of practice, but not to test best methods for putting standards into practice.
	Sampling can be used to test changes on a small scale; once improvements are agreed upon, additional data can be collected to verify results.
	Sampling is based on scientific principles and can satisfy many concerns about validity.

Developing and Testing Changes

Dx	Rx
No one can identify any change concepts that seem to apply to the project.	Change concepts are often useful for generating ideas for specific process changes. Sometimes, however, process changes can be identified first. Other sources of ideas for changes include brainstorming with the team, asking front-line staff and patients how they perceive the problem, and talking with other departments that may have similar process issues.
"We've tried to change things before, but nothing's worked."	Try to identify why previous efforts have failed: separate out whether the idea was flawed or the attempt to implement it ran into barriers.
	Emphasize that teams often learn more from failed tests than from successes.
	Remember that you'll be testing small changes first, so you'll be able to identify and adjust to problems as they come up.
Disagreement in the team about which changes to make first.	Remember that you'll be testing ideas for change, so you can learn quickly about which approaches seem to work.
	Plan to test several ideas at once.
	Use multivoting or other group process tools to make a quick decision about where to start; revisit decision after initial testing is completed.
"We're ready to identify changes we'd like to make, but we're afraid resources aren't available to us."	Share plans with your senior leader and get initial feedback; be specific about skills and/or resources needed.
	Test on a small scale to see if plans work before making a formal request for resources.
	Use small-scale data collection to minimize additional resources needed.
	Consider redefining the scope of the project if resources are an impediment; set initial aims for one department or one unit.

Dx	Rx
Changes may involve additional work for front-line individuals.	Ask senior management to provide additional resources for these individuals.
	Make the work a normal part of their day.
	Try to design changes that make everyday work easier rather than more difficult (e.g., consolidate different reporting forms).
	Identify opportunities to eliminate wasted efforts and unnecessary work.
	Make sure front-line staff are involved in designing changes.
Learning from PDSA cycles (tests of change) is often delayed for several weeks while waiting for tests to be completed.	Avoid large PDSA cycles which are often difficult to complete, absorbing time and energy. Cycles should be short but significant; test a big idea in a short time frame so that you can identify ways to improve or change the idea.
PDSA cycles are not connected to the aim.	In reflecting on what was learned from the test ("Study"), make sure it helps to achieve your aim.
	Plot outcome measures related to the aim over time.
PDSA cycles are not linked.	Connect "Study" phase of one cycle to "Plan" phase of the next one. Schedule specific times for reflecting on what was learned in carrying out cycles.

Team Composition and Functioning

Dx	Rx
Team meetings are unfocused and unproductive.	Revisit the basics: aim, measures, changes.
	Structure meetings around the PDSA cycles being tested.
	Visit other teams to see how their meetings work.
	Take advantage of the organization's resources for facilitators or training in team building.
	Consider changing the team membership if problems persist.
	Do a PDSA cycle that focuses on improving team functioning.
Meetings are too long.	Establish team rules regarding agenda-setting, timekeeping, roles and responsibilities.
	Make sure each meeting has a clear focus and objectives.
	Use PDSA cycles to test ways to shorten meetings.
	Use brief huddles between meetings to keep in touch and report on progress.
	Scale down the project based on time constraints.
The team does not meet regularly.	Investigate whether the issue is time or the lack of focus.
	If time is the issue, discuss resource availability with the senior leader; have other staff cover during meetings; have meetings before or after a shift.
	If lack of focus is the issue, revisit aims, and plan for testing changes.
	Schedule the next meeting at the beginning of each meeting.
	Use brief team huddles between meetings.

Dx	Rx
The team agrees on what is to be done but doesn't follow through.	Check the composition of the team; it should include systems, day-to-day, and technical leadership. A missing component can hamper implementation.
	Clarify the specific responsibilities of individuals and the time frames for completion.
	Investigate if the staff just don't have time to complete responsibilities; discuss with the team and with the senior leader.

Organizational Change Issues

Dx	Rx
Interdepartmental barriers to change.	Bring staff from other departments into the project; have staff from one department visit the other.
	Put patient care goals up front.
	Seek assistance of the senior leader.
Resistance to change.	Work with those who will work with you.
	Communicate goals and progress throughout the project.
	Building relationships is the key to winning over others; involving others in small tests of change can slowly help to redefine roles and relationships.
Physician resistance to change.	Identify one physician champion and work with that person. Use his or her improvement to convince others.
	Identify a nurse champion and include nurses that work with the physicians in your projects. The nurses can then work to help you influence those resistant physicians. Building nurses into the process can help with involving physicians.

Organizational Change Issues (continued)

Dx	Rx
Concerns about legal aspects of change.	Perform small tests of change based on good knowledge and experience.
	If it doesn't look or feel right, do not proceed with the test. Allow the implementer(s) of the actual change to stop the test if they deem it unwise to proceed (i.e., nursing personnel or respiratory therapy should feel free to not institute a protocol with which they feel uncomfortable). These situations should be viewed as additional learning opportunities.
Potential cost savings for your project seem small.	Costs add up. Calculate the potential cost savings throughout the organization over the course of a year.
No explicit approval for dedication of resources (time and/or people).	Propose that the team be a "skunkworks" to test the proposed improvements, and identify specific resources needed.
No visibility for project in the organization.	Write articles for the organization newsletter; use storyboards or posters to display progress.
Presence of other organizational changes such as mergers, downsizing, or reorganization.	Align the project with organizational goals.
	Stress staff involvement in changes, in contrast to top-down decisions.
	Focus on patient care as the ultimate goal.
	Emphasize connections among cost, productivity, patient care, and patient and staff satisfaction.
"That won't work here."	Build tension for change.
	Start small.
	Create opportunities for participation in change.
	Recruit resisters to suggest alternatives.
	Identify and publicize prior successful changes.
	Build momentum ("the theory of small wins").
	Communicate intentions and progress.

Dx	Rx
"We already have a change model."	The Model for Improvement is not meant to replace change models that organizations may be using but rather to accelerate improvement. The model creates tension to test ideas on a small scale rather than waiting until a solution is fully developed before action is taken.
Lack of senior leader support.	Align incentives: use data to show potential benefits of your work.
	Be realistic: offer senior leaders suggestions about highly leveraged uses of short amounts of their time.
	Focus on the concerns of the senior leader and help the leader understand how the project fits into institutional aims and vision.
	Request to be put on the agenda for the senior leadership group or the quality council.
	Identify an advocate who has the ear of the senior leader.
The senior leader is supportive, but there is little contact between the senior leader and the team.	Identify specific things you need from the senior leader and let the leader know what they are.
	Invite the senior leader to a team meeting.
	Keep the senior leader informed of your work; use e-mail, newsletter, briefings, etc.

In this section, you will find a variety of resources to help you make change in your organization:

BREAKTHROUGH SERIES ASSESSMENT

SUMMARY OF AIMS, CHANGES AND RESULTS

KEY CONTACTS

QUALITY IMPROVEMENT STORYBOARDS

IMPROVEMENT CYCLE WORKSHEET

ANNOTATED BIBLIOGRAPHY

Part 6

Resources for Reducing Delays and Waiting Times

Breakthrough Series Assessment

The Planning Group developed the following assessment tool to determine to what extent the Breakthrough Series Collaborative on Reducing Delays and Waiting Times met its stated goals.

Organizations engaged in making changes to achieve breakthrough improvement may find this tool useful in assessing their own progress.

The Breakthrough Series is built on the belief that organizations working together for 10 to 12 months, learning the latest scientific information available on improving a specific area of health care, and practical and effective means to put that knowledge into practice, can achieve breakthrough results.

The specific goal of the Collaborative on Reducing Delays and Waiting Times was clear and ambitious: 50% reduction in delays and waiting times within 12 months from June 1995 to June 1996. An assessment of 4 on the scale in Figure 6.1 would be consistent with that goal.

The scale integrates three dimensions:

- **Relative improvement:**
  The percent reduction in delays.
- **Actual level of performance achieved:**
  An organization that reduced delays from 40 minutes to 20 minutes would be rated higher than one that worked on the same system but reduced delays from 60 minutes to 30 minutes.
- **Size or complexity of the system:**
  Collaborative participants worked on systems of various sizes and complexities; progress with more complex systems is weighted in the ratings.

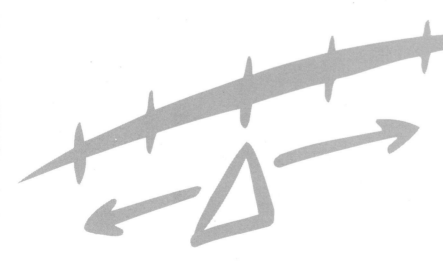

THE ASSESSMENT SCALE RATES ORGANIZATIONS ACCORDING TO FIVE CATEGORIES:

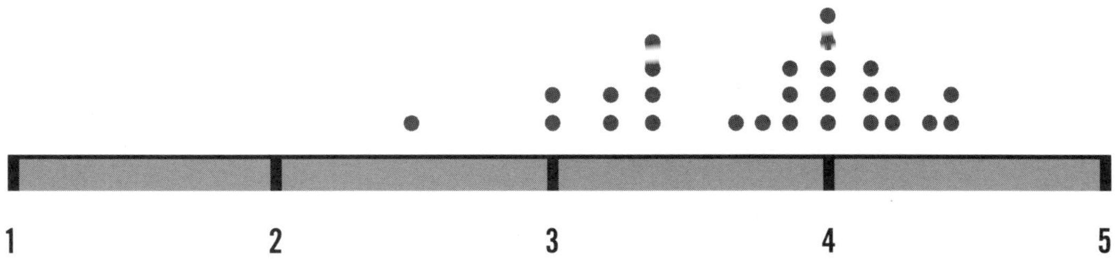

Collaborative Assessment, July 1996

Figure 6.1
ASSESSMENT: BREAKTHROUGH SERIES COLLABORATIVE ON REDUCING DELAYS AND WAITING TIMES (JUNE 1995–JUNE 1996)

Note:

- The scale is used as a visual analog scale, allowing a value anywhere along the scale.
- Each point represents one organization.
- The assessment is a consensus of the Planning Group and the Collaborative organizations.

1. Nonstarter

The organization attended the first Learning Session of the Collaborative but dropped out shortly thereafter.

2. Activity but no changes

The organization actively engaged in the effort, but its initiatives do not include any changes. For example, it conducted a literature search or raised awareness about the project in the organization.

3. Modest improvement

Anecdotal evidence about rational changes.

Evidence of improvements (10% to 30% reduction in delay) in a localized process; for example, operating room turnaround time.

Early indications of improvement of a large system; for example, major redesign of clinic flow.

4. Significant progress

Reduction in delay for a major subsystem of 40% to 50%; for example, admission to the inpatient unit from the emergency department or the patient acute care unit.

Reduction in delay at the system level for a cohort of patients of 40% to 50%; for example, extremity patients in the emergency department or orthopedic surgery patients.

5. Outstanding, sustainable results

Reduction in delay at the system level of 50% or more; for example, all office waits or all surgeries.

Achieved levels are at the leading edge.

Summary of Aims, Changes, and

The organizations who participated in the Breakthrough Series Collaborative on Reducing Delays and Waiting Times worked together for 12 months beginning in June 1995 to achieve breakthrough improvement.

The following chart summarizes their work: each organization's aim, the major changes they made, and the results they achieved. The organizations are grouped according to four areas of primary focus: emergency department, surgery, clinics and physicians' offices, and access to care.

Results

Reducing Delays in the Emergency Department

ORGANIZATION	Chester County Hospital West Chester, PA	Children's Hospital Boston, MA
AIM	Reduce perceived and actual waiting time in the ED.	Reduce waiting time for ED patients, especially asthma patients and nonurgent febrile infants.
CHANGES	Develop Med Express system: separate process for nonurgent patients. Develop Be-a-Bed-Ahead system: pulls patients from ED to receiving unit.	Implement asthma clinical practice guideline, including establishing standards for nebulizer administration, reorganizing supplies, obtaining peak flow meters for triage area, and improving patient education materials and communication to primary care provider. Redesign patient flow in ED, break up exam room bottlenecks by using the inner waiting room for patients in the process of care. Move patients from triage directly into an exam room for evaluation and bedside registration, when exam rooms and staff are available.
RESULTS	Reduced Med Express total process time from 98 minutes to 39 minutes. All patients in ED seen by a physician within 39 minutes of arrival (versus 66 minutes in May 1995). ED patients moving to inpatient units wait 61 minutes (versus 88 minutes in May 1995).	Decreased median time for treatment initiation for asthmatics by 50% (from 50 minutes to 24 minutes). Decreased average time from triage to blood work initiation for non-urgent febrile infants from 105 minutes to 40 minutes. Time from triage to time seen by a physician in the ED averages 18 minutes.

Reducing Delays in the Emergency Department

ORGANIZATION	**Christ Hospital** Jersey City, NJ	**Columbia Wesley Medical Center** Wichita, KS
AIM	Reduce delays for patients being admitted to telemetry unit from ED.	Reduce elapsed time from triage to treatment for ED patients.
CHANGES	Improve utilization of telemetry beds. Direct nursing-to-nursing admission request from ED to telemetry unit.	Initiate Quick Admit process: minimize information needed for registration at triage and defer completion of registration process until patient is in the treatment area. Assess vital signs in triage. Triage nurse contacts physician for preapproval as required. Use triage assessment as basic assessment for nonurgent patients.
RESULTS	Reduced inpatient telemetry length of stay from 5.8 days to 3.8 days and related waits for admission from ED to telemetry from two hours (in October 1995) to 30 minutes or less (in June 1996).	Reduced average time from triage to treatment from 30 minutes to 20 minutes.

Northwest Covenant Medical Center Denville, NJ	**SSM Health Care System/ St. Francis Hospital & Health Center** Blue Island, IL
Reduce waiting time for ED patients, and reduce turnaround time for lab results.	Reduce time from physician discharge order to patient discharge.
Redesign process for ordering x-rays for abdominal, skull, rib, and lower back patients.	Place chart racks on all units for easy identification of patients to be discharged. Document all discharge instructions on discharge sheet at the time the intervention takes place, rather than waiting until day of discharge. Transport patients to their cars using Patient Care Unit personnel, rather than waiting for centralized transportation department. Place discharge instruction form on front of the patient chart; encourage physicians to complete their portion of the discharge instruction sheet rather than having nursing copy information from the medical record to the form. Incorporate patient education and expected LOS in care pathway protocols, helping patients and families anticipate and prepare for discharge.
Pilot-tested changes and achieved reduced delays in selected groups of patients.	Reduced average waiting time for discharge of inpatients from 2.7 hours to 1.2 hours.

Reducing Delays in the Emergency Department

ORGANIZATION	**SSM Health Care System/St. Mary's Health Center** St. Louis, MO	**St. Joseph's Mercy Hospitals and Health Services** Clinton Township, MI
AIM	Reduce total length of stay in ED.	Reduce length of visit for patients with simple extremity injuries requiring radiology studies.
CHANGES	Initiate Quick Admit process: minimize information needed to generate ED records and registration number and defer completion of registration process until patient is in treatment area.	Establish protocol for patient flow through ED. Reduce number of patient handoffs. Enter x-ray order sooner. Develop pull system for patients by x-ray technicians. Patient has one encounter with physician.
RESULTS	Reduced triage to treatment time from 45 minutes to 15 minutes or less over three-month period.	Reduced length of visit for extremity patients from 130 minutes in September 1995 to less than 80 minutes in April 1996.

York Health System
York, PA

Reduce delays in bed placement for patients being admitted from the ED.

Improve utilization of intensive care, transitional, and telemetry beds.

Admit directly to the admitting unit.

Admitting unit assigns beds.

Develop a Be-a-Bed-Ahead system: pull system from receiving unit for both ED and post-anesthesia care unit (PACU) patients.

Decreased median holding time for patients being transferred to all inpatient units from 60 minutes in January 1996 to 36 minutes in June 1996.

Reducing Delays in Surgery

ORGANIZATION	**Beth Israel Deaconess Medical Center–East Campus** Boston, MA	**Beth Israel Deaconess Medical Center–West Campus** Boston, MA
AIM	Reduce delays in surgery process, including preoperative testing and transfer of patients from PACU to inpatient units following surgery.	Reduce delays on day of surgery.
CHANGES	Create a flexible "first available provider" order process for preoperative testing, use telephonic screening for most ASA Class I and Class II patients. Substitute fax report for oral nurse-to-nurse report for patients transferred from PACU to inpatient unit.	Utilize custom packs, customize case cart by surgeon and case type. Do instrument set-up, patient preparation and drape, surgeon scrub in parallel. Decrease utilization of invasive lines, insert lines in holding area. Set up in advance for next case, use "Swing Room."
RESULTS	Reduced total delay for preoperative testing from 58 minutes to 21 minutes. Reduced average delays for PACU patients by 64% (from 66 minutes to 23 minutes) and reduced percent of patients delayed from 51% to 7%.	Reduced utilization of PA Catheters by 50% in CABG population. *Comparing a 3-month period in 1995 to 1996:* Reduced room turnaround time by 11 minutes. Reduced arrival time to incision time for first vascular case by 8 minutes or 17.9%. Improved "in room" time of first vascular case by 10 minutes or 16.6%.

Dartmouth-Hitchcock Medical Center Lebanon, NH	**Sewickley Valley Hospital** Sewickley, PA
Streamline preadmission testing process for surgical patients, using computerized patient self-assessment tool.	Reduce delays in surgical services: all outpatients ready for incision within 90 minutes after arrival in outpatient surgery.
Develop Healthquiz: patient administered, computerized anesthesia assessment program. Complete facility renovations. Implement changes in patient education, nursing and anesthesia consult process, and provider education.	Redesign surgery department processes and staff responsibilities to synchronize all tasks to time of incision, including anesthesia preparation and assessment, room and instrument set-up, transport of patients, and surgeon arrival.
Patients are now accommodated on walk-in basis, requiring only one visit for surgical clearance. Reduced patient waiting time to see a provider to less than 15 minutes 80% of the time. Decreased operating room turn-around time by three minutes on average, even though anesthesia sees majority of patients for the first time on morning of surgery. Reduced average first case "in room" time by 20 minutes from June 1995 to June 1996. Reduced cancellations due to "medically not clear" from 1.2% in June 1995 to 0.01% in June 1996.	Reduced delays in surgery starts from 83% of the time in January 1996 to 33% of the time in July 1996.

Reducing Waiting Time in Clinics and Physicians' Offices

ORGANIZATION	**Covenant Healthcare System, Inc.** Milwaukee, WI	**Deborah Heart and Lung Center** Browns Mills, NJ
AIM	Redesign registration process to allow patient to register once in the system and go directly to area providing needed service; reduce rework and cost in revenue management cycle.	Reduce waiting time for patients coming to Ambulatory Services Center (ASC) for outpatient testing.
CHANGES	Eliminate duplicative records. Implement one registration for all sites of care. Maintain accurate, available data. Create ability to transfer data from site-to-site. Reduce number of signatures obtained. Reshape demand for services. Send patients directly to service area.	Restructure physician services in cardiology to create time for more clinics. Add new clinics during less-utilized afternoon times. Create nurse/physician teams to provide continuity of care. Develop and implement universal patient history form to standardize database. Eliminate redundant clinical assessments by nurses and physicians.
RESULTS	Decreased average waiting time for patient registration at pilot hospital by 50%, from just under eight minutes in December 1995 to less than four minutes in December 1996.	Decreased average time for outpatient cardiology visit from 198 minutes to 139 minutes and decreased average waiting time from 105 minutes to 62 minutes. Decreased time patient spends with nursing staff from 28 minutes to 12 minutes. Decreased time to next appointment in cardiology from 21 days to 1 day.

Franciscan Skemp Healthcare – Mayo Health System
La Crosse, WI

Reduce delays in access to internal medicine appointments, and reduce waiting times during visit.

Relocate physicians' offices to facilitate communication and sharing of rooms.

Set up mail sorting system to reduce physician distractions during clinic time.

Pull charts one day in advance of appointment.

Change physician-call procedure.

Nurses and triage nurse coordinate physician availability for same-day appointments.

Modify scheduling.

Utilize extra nurse for triage line during peak times.

Use waiting list for patients to get earlier appointments when they become available.

Preliminary data on selected physicians shows improved access and reduced waiting times in clinic.

Reducing Waiting Time in Clinics and Physicians' Offices

ORGANIZATION	**HealthPartners** Minneapolis, MN
AIM	Reduce total waiting time to no longer than 15 minutes.
CHANGES	Schedule more complex patients at end of session. Redistribute nonpatient care tasks to nonphysician staff. Shift delay from exam room to lobby. Use exam room waiting time for preventive services. Use morning huddles for staff to review schedule. Communicate on-time status among physician/nurse/receptionist. Standardize stocking of rooms. Synchronize timing of tasks to appointment time: complete lab and x-ray tests, with results recorded on chart. Use guidelines to assess need for physician appointment. Schedule additional appointment for unexpected needs when clinically appropriate. Identify systemwide applications of changes.
RESULTS	Decreased average waiting times from 20 minutes to less than 12 minutes. Identified systemwide applications.

UNITYChoice Health Plan Des Moines, IA	**University of Michigan Medical Center** Ann Arbor, MI
Reduce waiting time for patients at selected clinics.	Reduce waiting time in urology clinic.
Use physician assistants in primary care. Provide information on self-care. Give the patient a specific "when to arrive" time rather than the traditional appointment time, in order to better synchronize the patient's arrival with the provider's schedule.	Synchronize first patient arrival with physician arrival. Use realistic time slots for procedures. Redesign schedule to put new patient (unpredictable) visits first and return (predictable) visits later in the day.
Measured difference between scheduled appointment time and first greeting in clinic, time from greeting to nurse contact, and time from nurse contact to physician contact at selected clinics.	Reduced waiting time for patients seeing selected physicians by 12%. Reduced variability in length of visit by 35% for selected physicians. Reduced annualized overtime costs by 59%.

Increasing Access to Care

ORGANIZATION	**Cambridge Hospital** Cambridge, MA	**Department of Veterans Affairs Medical Center** New Orleans, LA
AIM	Decrease delay between desired and actual primary care visit.	Reduce delays for patients in scheduling visits with subspecialists.
CHANGES	Schedule routine health visits by month of birth and diagnosis. Offer alternative service to patients who reschedule routinely. Use available slots during resident sessions for urgent care with minimal triage. Adjust schedule to match provider availability to demand. Add urgent care slots for all providers. Provide specialized education services for diabetic patients.	Decrease new patient visits, improve productivity and performance of clinic, and eliminate unnecessary follow-up visits. *Specific changes include:* Eliminate appointments more than six months out. Add extra day of clinic; abolish subspecialty clinics. Match existing workload. Limit access to scheduling system to clinic clerks. Utilize electronic urology health summary. Use guidelines to determine appropriateness for clinic visit. Discharge no-shows.
RESULTS	Achieved initial drop in "number of days to third next appointment" as measure of access to primary care appointments.	Reduced average time to wait for urology clinic appointment from over 150 days to less than 50 days; reduced average wait for ophthalmology clinic appointment from just under 200 days to less than 100 days.

GHMA Medical Centers/HealthPartners of Southern Arizona Tucson, AZ	**HealthSystem Minnesota** St. Louis Park, MN
Improve access to primary care providers.	Increase delivery of essential preventive care by delivering services at every patient encounter (thereby decreasing demand for yearly physicals and increasing acute care access).
Match high-demand days to provider availability. Identify high-utilizer patients for case management intervention. Distribute patient education manual. Develop simplified scheduling at pilot site. Identify and eliminate bottlenecks in back office.	Implement screening guidelines. Develop and integrate visit planning materials. Empower support staff to schedule needed services (e.g., standing orders). Develop automated computer system preventive care labels. Use phone care for follow-up of risk assessments. Develop system for measuring and reporting provider performance. Centralize chart for recording adult essential services, immunizations, medications, allergies, smoking status, and chronic problems.
Decreased average wait for same-day appointments, routine physicals, and routine appointments.	Improved delivery of essential preventive care from 4% to 46% in one department.

Increasing Access to Care

ORGANIZATION	**MetroHealth** Indianapolis, IN	**Virginia Mason Medical Center** Seattle, WA
AIM	Improve access to primary care appointments.	Reduce delays in accessing primary care.
CHANGES	Give reminders for recheck appointments due after two months in lieu of scheduling an appointment. Establish hypertension clinic. Increase early morning access.	Physicians make a time commitment to maintain appointment availability. Balance volumes and work loads. Decrease unnecessary variation in appointment types and lengths. Distribute tasks appropriately. Create a team and foster inter-dependency. Allocate resources by volume of work.
RESULTS	Increased availability of all types of primary care appointments from 51% in August 1995 to over 90% in June 1996. Increased percentage of pediatric patients offered routine appointments within one week of request from 41% to 100%.	Reduced average wait for a routine (return) physical exam for an established patient from 42 days to 13 days.

Watson Clinic LLP
Lakeland, FL

Increase access by having appropriate number of correct appointment types available to match patient demand.

Establish Advice Center.

Use open scheduling system with established physician.

Match capacity to demand by adding new physician.

Establish regional clinics.

Establish nurse-run clinic.

Reduced the number of days until next available appointment for a physical from 40 days to 26.5 days.

Key Contacts

Collaborative Chair and Director

Thomas W. Nolan, PhD
Statistician
Collaborative Chair

Associates in Process Improvement
1110 Bonifant Street, Suite 420
Silver Springs, MD 20910
Tel: (301) 589-7981

Marie W. Schall, MA
Collaborative Director

319 Flynn Avenue
Moorestown, NJ 08057
Tel: (609) 778-0591
FAX: (609) 727-7563
E-Mail: mschall@ix.netcom.com

Beth Israel Deaconess Medical Center – East Campus
330 Brookline Avenue, KS132
Boston, MA 02215

Daryl Juran
Internal Quality Improvement Consultant
Training and Development
Tel: (617) 667-3785
FAX: (617) 667-7198
E-Mail: djuran@bih.harvard.edu

Beth Israel Deaconess Medical Center – West Campus
One Deaconess Road
Boston, MA 02215

Nancy Wilkinson, RN
Senior Staff Consultant
Tel: (617) 632-8269
FAX: (617) 632-7887
E-Mail: nwilkins@nedhmail.
nedh.harvard.edu

Cambridge Hospital
1493 Cambridge Street
Cambridge, MA 02139

Stephen Oakley
Business Manager, Primary and
Family Health
Tel: (617) 498-1571
FAX: (617) 498-1506
E-Mail: soakley@std.world.com

Chester County Hospital
701 East Marshall Street
West Chester, PA 19380

Kay Holbrook
Director, Case Management
Tel: (610) 431-5137
FAX: (610) 430-2941
E-Mail: chesterk@ix.netcom.com

Children's Hospital
300 Longwood Avenue
Boston, MA 02115

Fran Damian, RN, MS
Director, Nursing and Patient Services
Tel: (617) 355-5944
FAX: (617) 355-6625
E-Mail: Damian@al.tch.harvard.edu.@SMTP

Patricia A. Rutherford, RN, MS
Nursing/Patient Services Director
Tel: (617) 355-7591
FAX: (617) 734-3458
E-Mail: rutherford@a1.tch.harvard.edu

Christ Hospital
176 Palisade Avenue
Jersey City, NJ 07306

Maureen LaParo
Quality Director
Tel: (201) 795-5758
FAX: (201) 418-7068
E-Mail: Maureen@LaParo.com

Columbia Wesley Medical Center
550 North Hillside, Suite 104
Wichita, KS 67214

Linda J. Mild, RN, MS
Senior Vice President, Clinical Services
Tel: (316) 688-2050
FAX: (316) 688-7093
E-Mail: lynmild@ix.netcom.com

Covenant Healthcare System, Inc.
1126 South 70th Street
Milwaukee, WI 53214-0970

Penny J. Goodyear, RN, MSN
Regional Director
Tel: (414) 456-2336
FAX: (414) 456-2363

Dartmouth-Hitchcock Medical Center
One Medical Center Drive
Lebanon, NH 03756

Ronald Sliwinski
Vice President
Tel: (603) 650-8169
FAX: (603) 650-8765

Deborah Heart and Lung Center
200 Trenton Road
Browns Mills, NJ 08015

Charles Dennis, MD
Chairman, Department of Cardiology
Tel: (609) 735-2905
FAX: (609) 893-6038
E-Mail: cdennis748@aol.com

Department of Veterans Affairs Medical Center
1601 Perdido Street
New Orleans, LA 70146

Harry Pigman, MD
Deputy Chief of Staff
Tel: (504) 568-0811
FAX: (504) 589-5211
E-Mail: pigman@neworleans.va.gov

Franciscan Skemp Healthcare – Mayo Health System
700 West Avenue, South
La Crosse, WI 54601

Jean Krause, BS, RRA
Director, Quality Improvement
Tel: (608) 791-9711
FAX: (608) 791-9429
E-Mail: jkrause@fsh.mayo.edu

GHMA Medical Centers/HealthPartners of Southern Arizona
2945 West Ina Road
Tucson, AZ 85741

Madeleine Lucas
Staff Development Coordinator
Tel: (520) 751-3616
FAX: (520) 297-0668

Group Health Cooperative of Puget Sound
950 Pacific Avenue, Suite 900
Tacoma, WA 98402

Glenda Anderson
Service Quality Manager
Tel: (206) 383-6261
FAX: (206) 383-5981
E-Mail: anderson.g@ghc.org

Sharon Linton, MBA
(Formerly with Group Health Cooperative of Puget Sound)
Tel: (206) 649-7704
FAX: (206) 383-5981

HealthPartners
8100 34th Avenue South, PO Box 1309
Minneapolis, MN 55440-1309

Kathy Monahan-Rial
Manager of Clinic Systems for Development and Support
Tel: (612) 883-5832
FAX: (612) 883-5880
E-Mail: kathy.m.monahanria@
healthpartners.com

HealthSystem Minnesota
3800 Park Nicollet Boulevard
St. Louis Park, MN 55416

Sharon Reiter
Director, Patient Access Services
Tel: (612) 993-3309
FAX: (612) 993-5758

Kaiser Permanente Colorado
10350 East Dakota Avenue
Denver, CO 80231-1314

Robert Lederer, MD
Assistant to Medical Director,
Best Practices
Tel: (303) 344-7684
FAX: (303) 344-7208
E-Mail: bobleder@ix.netcom.com

MetroHealth
Methodist Medical Towers
1633 North Capitol, Suite 912
Indianapolis, IN 46202

Eric Bindewald, MD
Medical Director
Tel: (317) 929-1775
FAX: (317) 929-2474
E-Mail: ebindewald@usa.pipeline.com

Northwest Covenant Medical Center
25 Pocono Road
Denville, NJ 07834

Michael Siman, PhD
Director, Research and Evaluation
Tel: (201) 625-7093
FAX: (201) 625-3619
E-Mail: MLSiman@aol.com

Sewickley Valley Hospital
720 Blackburn Road
Sewickley, PA 15143

Marcia Cifrulak, RN
Staff Nurse, Operating Room
Tel: (412) 749-7530
FAX: (412) 749-7543

Marilyn Rudolph, RN
(Formerly with Sewickley Valley Hospital)
Director of Performance
Improvement Collaboratives
VHA Pennsylvania, Inc.
Tel: (412) 922-9124
FAX: (412) 922-1672

SSM Health Care System
477 N. Lindbergh Boulevard
St. Louis, MO 63141

Barbara Spreadbury, RRA
Corporate Director
Quality Resource Center
Tel: (314) 994-7747
FAX: (314) 994-7900
E-Mail: bspreadbury@ssmhcs.com

SSM Health Care System/St. Francis Hospital & Health Center
12935 South Gregory Street
Blue Island, IL 60406

Pat Sutton
Manager, Social Services
Tel: (708) 597-2000, ext. 5267
FAX: (708) 597-7508

SSM Health Care System/St. Mary's Health Center
6420 Clayton Road
St. Louis, MO 63117

Marianne Fournie
Patient Care Manager
Emergency Department
Tel: (314) 768-8316
FAX: (314) 768-8011

St. Joseph's Mercy Hospitals and Health Services
15855 Nineteen Mile Road
Clinton Township, MI 48038

Jan Bolton
QA Coordinator/Patient Services
Tel: (810) 263-2631
FAX: (810) 263-2614
E-Mail: jmbolton@ix.netcom.com

UNITYChoice Health Plan
6th & Grand Avenue
Des Moines, IA 50309

Kirk Phillips
Medical Research Consultant
Tel: (515) 237-6634

University of Michigan Medical Center
1500 East Medical Center Drive
MPB D5101
Ann Arbor, MI 48109-0718

Linda Larin, MBA
Associate Hospital Administrator
Tel: (313) 764-3507
FAX: (313) 936-9616
E-Mail: llarin@umich.edu

VHA Pennsylvania, Inc.
415 Holiday Drive, Bldg. 1
Pittsburgh, PA 15220

Patricia A. Banaszak
Vice President of Quality
Clinical Development
Tel: (412) 922-9124
FAX: (412) 922-1672
E-Mail: banaszak@ix.netcom.com

Virginia Mason Medical Center
1100 Ninth Avenue
PO Box 900, M/S GBADM
Seattle, WA 98111

Carolyn Cone
Project Manager
Tel: (206) 583-6528
FAX: (206) 223-6976
E-Mail: admc1c@vmmcis.vmmc.org

Watson Clinic LLP
1600 Lakeland Hills Boulevard
Lakeland, FL 33805

Melinda Harrison
Director, Clinical Services
Tel: (941) 680-7922
FAX: (941) 680-7978
E-Mail: xfsc23a@prodigy.com

York Health System
1001 South George Street
York, PA 17405

Connie Sixta, RN, MSN
Vice President, Operations
Tel: (717) 851-2754
FAX: (717) 851-3020
E-Mail: csixta@yorkhospital.edu

Quality Improvement Storyboards

The following guidelines are used by organizations in the Breakthrough Series to prepare storyboards. Storyboards are a valued tool of the Breakthrough Series for effectively presenting an organization's work to a variety of audiences—to other organizations within each collaborative, to the larger audience at each National Congress, and to the home audience within each organization.

PURPOSE

A storyboard is a presentation of a project in a poster fashion for others to examine. Its purpose is to communicate a story—the story of the work that has been performed.

GOAL

The goal of a storyboard presentation is to capture the reader's attention quickly and to communicate the desired information clearly and succinctly.

Guiding Principles:

Storyboards should tell the truth without fudging. There are three classifications of storyboards, each of which has a particular value and addresses different lessons learned:

- those that display success in reaching the organization's goals;
- those that display good progress in reaching the organization's goals;
- those representing organizations that were unable to achieve significant progress toward the goals, but learned critical lessons in the process. These stories are as important as others and should be tailored to describe obstacles to change.

Key Characteristics:

Creativity should be used in poster design, but care must be taken to make the presentations understandable in a brief period of time. Complex charts or tables will diminish the viewer's ability to comprehend the content rapidly, and should be avoided. Likewise, presenting too much information overwhelms the reader and diminishes the impact of the presentation.

- Design for ease of comprehension and readability.
- Include only critical information.
- Keep it simple.
- Make purpose of the investigation readily apparent.
- Describe interventions concisely.
- Display data over time using control charts.
- Outline conclusions based upon data.
- Present plans for implementation or further investigation.

Sample Storyboard Outline:

1. **Title and Introduction:** Briefly state title and organization name. Give a brief background for the project, including simple data illustrating the problem.

2. **Aim:** State the goals of the project succinctly.

3. **List PDSA Cycles:** In concert with displaying of PDSA cycle dates on the data chart(s), briefly list (in several words) the change or intervention corresponding to each cycle. For the two or three most important PDSA cycles, give a more detailed description (a few sentences) of the specific intervention(s). Try to group cycles into major categories (or ramps), as shown in the examples in Part 2. Only include cycles in which a test of change resulted in concrete action. For example, do not list meetings, presentations, or preparation of materials as separate cycles.

4. **Plot Data:** Using a control chart(s) or other appropriate charts, display the data chronologically. Label the chart using arrows to show the time frame of each cycle, including the next cycle planned, thereby displaying multiple cycles on one chart.

5. **Conclusions:** In a few sentences, describe the results of this work.

6. **Next Steps or Future Plans:** In a few sentences, describe any plans for the next few cycles.

Improving Access to Outpatient Medical Services

SAMPLE STORYBOARD

GHMA MEDICAL CENTERS/HEALTHPARTNERS OF SOUTHERN ARIZONA

Background and Introduction

Demand far exceeded capacity for outpatient medical care at GHMA in July 1995. Our data on access to primary care providers and efficiency of outpatient services as measured by the need for employees to work overtime hours demonstrated:

Waiting time until a patient could schedule an appointment:

Average wait was > 20 days for "same-day" care.

Average wait was > 45 days for a routine appointment.

Efficiency of outpatient services:

23 overtime hours/2 weeks were required by staff to meet scheduling demands in the NorthWest Family Medicine Department.

We believe the problem with access to our primary care providers compromised our ability to deliver consistent high-quality care. In addition, increased costs were incurred since patients were often asked to use urgent care centers or emergency departments for their acute care.

Aim

We sought to improve outpatient access to primary care providers by meeting or exceeding guidelines for outpatient access as set by our organization.

These standards include:

Average waiting time for same-day care: 1 day

represents a 90% reduction in waiting times for same-day visits.

Average waiting time for routine visit: 21 days

represents a > 50% reduction in waiting times for routine visits.

In addition, it was our intent to provide patients with a requested appointment at the time requested in a hassle-free manner.

Methods

We focused on the following areas:

I. Changing Demand
Implement alternative means of caring for patients who are high utilizers of outpatient services by providing educational programs and alternate ways of receiving medical advice.

II. Changing Scheduling Process
Restructure our scheduling procedure to a semiflexible system in which a combination of visit types are reserved for same-day and routine care.

III. Communication
Understand patient needs by conducting surveys and change the culture within our organization to continually strive to meet those needs.

IV. Processes of Patient Care
Examine the processes of care within our patient care areas for bottlenecks and change our processes to eliminate those bottlenecks.

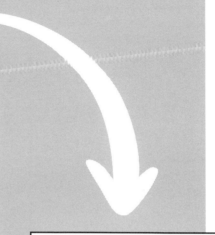

Outcome Measure

Changes in outpatient access will be measured by examining the waiting time for the next available appointment for same day care and routine care using two sample physicians. Measurements will be made one day per week during the study period.

Change Cycles

I. Changing Demand

Identify high-demand days and match providers' clinical time to the demand on these days.	Fall 1995
Develop criteria to define a "high-maintenance patient" or a "high-utilizer patient"and select high-utilizer patients for case management intervention.	12/95
Improve patient education by using Healthwise manuals.	12/95–2/96
Establish plans to work down the backlog.	1/96
Future Cycles:	4/96

- Initiate use of Healthwise manuals at other centers.
- Implement the Personal Health Improvement Program to meet the needs of "high-utilizer" patients.

CONTINUES...

II. Changing Scheduling Process

Develop new format for scheduling.	12/95
Prepare scheduling guidelines and training materials, present to staff, obtain feedback, and revise.	12/95 - 2/96
Train receptionists and test simplified scheduling.	3/96
Future Cycle: Implement simplified scheduling at other centers.	

III. Communication

Develop and implement a patient satisfaction survey.	12/95
Develop methods to increase productivity with input from the administration and staff.	1/96

IV. Processes of Patient Care

Determine bottlenecks in back office and implement changes to improve patient flow.	12/95
Implement Unit Associate position and shift clerical demand from nurse and provider to Unit Associate.	1/96

Results

Implementation of a new scheduling system had significant impact on improving patient's access to primary care. The average wait for routine appointments is also improving steadily.

Routine Visit Waiting Times

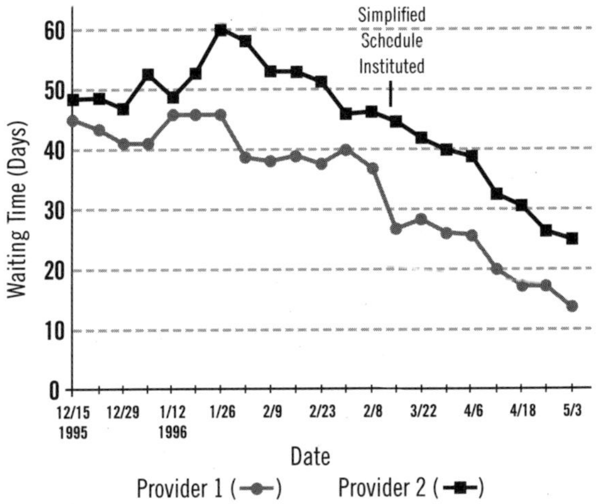

Note: Provider 2 is the only female physician at her center and is in high demand by female patients for routine physical and pelvic examinations. An additional female physician is being added to that center.

Results (continued)

The average wait for same-day care was reduced from more than 20 days to 1 day (i.e., within 24 hours), a [illegible] improvement.

Same-Day Care Waiting Times

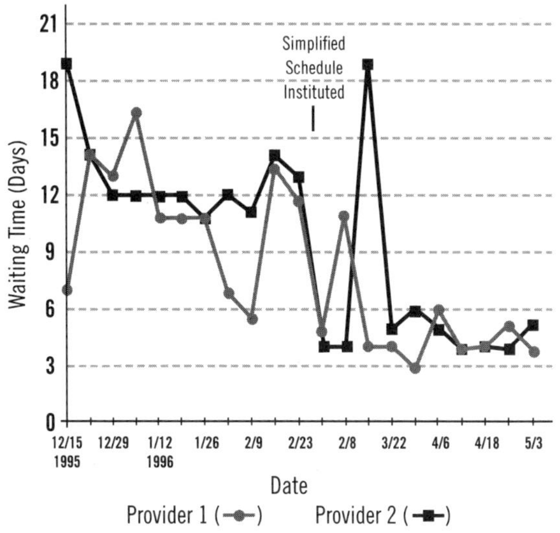

Next Steps

Plans include the following:

- Identify leaders among management and provider staff to take ownership of the numerous processes.
- Begin disseminating this work into other areas of our health system.
- Continue to reshape demand by implementing patient education/intervention programs.
- Additional analysis of work flow in physicians' offices to improve efficiency.
- Develop a better understanding of the demand for outpatient services by tracking and measuring key elements.

Improvement Cycle Worksheet

Organizations in the Collaborative on Reducing Delays and Waiting Times documented and reported their work on testing changes using the following format. Each improvement cycle worksheet documents one Plan-Do-Study-Act cycle.

BREAKTHROUGH SERIES COLLABORATIVE TO REDUCE DELAYS AND WAIT TIMES

Improvement Cycle Worksheet

Organization: Children's Hospital, Boston

Team Leader: Pat Rutherford Date: Sept. 15

Cycle #: 1 Began: Aug. 31 Completed: Sept. 9

PLAN:

Objective of this cycle: To test the changes in the new documentation package for the Short Stay Unit.

What additional information will we need to take action? Determine what refinements are needed to make the forms functional for doctors and nurses.

Details (Who, What, Where, When, How):

Who - doctors and nurses will use the new documentation forms

What - consolidate admission assessment and MD work-up, order sheet and medication schedule, flowsheet and progress notes, and discharge information

Where - 10 beds utilized for SSU patients

When - from August 31 through September 9

Why - to simplify documentation (reduce redundancies, eliminate unnecessary steps, combine components)

What do we predict will happen? Efficiencies in documentation will be achieved; new documentation at the bedside may be confusing to those not on the unit.

DO:

Was the cycle carried out as planned? Yes, but some minor changes in the documentation forms were made immediately (instead of waiting for the complete trial).

What did we observe that was not part of our plan? Obtained feedback on a daily basis.

SAMPLE IMPROVEMENT CYCLE WORKSHEET

PAGE 1

PAGE 2

***STUDY*:**

Methods of analysis: Noted experiences and feedback of nurses and doctors who had used the new documentation forms; qualitative analysis to ascertain common problems.

How did or didn't the results of this cycle agree with the predictions that we made earlier?

Problems did arise for those outside of the unit.

Documentation was more efficient and streamlined.

Staff needed to acquire new habits of charting at the bedside.

List what new knowledge we gained by this cycle.

1. Community MDs and attendings did not know where to find the chart and where to chart progress notes.
2. Nurses and MDs needed to write on the assessment form at the same time.
3. There wasn't enough light in the patient rooms to chart at the bedside.

***ACT*:**

List the actions we will take as a result of this cycle.

1. Nurses and house staff to orient attendings and community pediatricians to the documentation changes.
2. Separate MD work-up from nursing assessment form.
3. At night, put the documentation on a bedside table outside the patient's room.

Are there forces in our organziation that will help or hinder these changes? Explain.

Need for clinicians to chart at the bedside - met some resistance.

A computerized medical record would enhance the successful implementation of these changes (not in the near future).

Objectives of our next cycle:

Test the modification for 2 weeks.

The aim of the team from Children's Hospital in Boston, MA was to reduce delays for patients in the short stay unit. This sample worksheet reports on a test of a new documentation package for the short stay unit. The organization developed the package (Plan), then tested it in 10 beds on the short stay unit (Do). The team's study of the effects of the change (Study) indicated several ways in which the package could be improved. The team proceeded to make modifications and refinements (Act) before eventually implementing the change on the entire short stay unit.

Annotated Bibliography

GENERAL LITERATURE ON QUALITY IMPROVEMENT

Berwick D. Continuous improvement as an ideal in health care. *N Engl J Med.* 1989;320:53-56.

A classic, one of the first published calls for systems thinking in clinical care.

Berwick DM, Godfrey AB, Roessner J. *Curing Health Care: New Strategies for Quality Improvement.* San Francisco: Jossey-Bass Publishers; 1990.

This book explains how healthcare leaders can apply methods of modern quality management in their organizations to improve efficiency and safety, achieve new breakthroughs in performance, reduce costs, and help reshape our troubled healthcare system. Drawing on the experiences and lessons of the National Demonstration Project on Quality Improvement in Health Care, the authors show how quality management techniques adopted from industry can be applied to solve specific problems in health care.

Eye on Improvement. Boston: Institute for Healthcare Improvement.

This newsletter, which publishes abstracts of articles from about 50 different journals in 24 yearly issues, is one good way to keep up with the rapidly expanding literature in CQI. (Editorial office: P.O. Box 38100, Cleveland, Ohio 44138; 1-800-895-4951).

Gaucher EJ, Coffey RJ. *Total Quality in Health Care: From Theory to Practice.* San Francisco: Jossey-Bass Publishers; 1993.

As the title suggests, the authors link theory to practice in CQI, using their experience in implementing quality management at the University of Michigan Medical Center. Chapter 7 explores the role of physicians.

Goldfield N, Nash DB, eds. *Providing Quality Care: The Challenge to Clinicians.* 2nd ed. Philadelphia: American College of Physicians; 1995.

Provides a summary of the work of leading researchers in health services research, with an editorial commentary at the end of each chapter.

GENERAL LITERATURE ON DELAYS, WAITING TIMES AND ACCESS ISSUES

Carlson JG. Just-in-time approach to systemwide efficiency and quality borrows from industrial techniques. *Strateg Healthc Excell.* 1993;6(2):9–12.

This article reviews the basics in management for optimization of customer service in health care.

Chapman SN, Carmel JI. Demand/capacity management in health care: An application of yield management. *Health Care Manage Rev.* 1992;17:45–54.

Yield management is a system to match demand with constrained capacity that is used in many non-healthcare industries. This article describes the application of yield management techniques in health care.

Fries JF. Health care demand management. *Med Interface.* 1994;7(3):55–58.

Healthcare organizations must learn how to manage the demands for their services in order to provide better services while lowering costs.

Fries JF, Koop CE, Beadle CE, et al. Reducing health care costs by reducing the need and demand for medical services. The Health Project Consortium. *New Engl J Med.* 1993;329:321–325.

The Health Project Consortium provides a detailed discussion of demand management. The report proposes that wider use of preventive care would control the growth of medical expenditures and make patients healthier at the same time.

Hall RW. *Queuing Methods for Services and Manufacturing.* Englewood Cliffs, NJ: Prentice-Hall; 1991.

This book provides basic statistical methodology for queuing theory.

Langley G, Nolan K, Nolan T, Norman C, Provost L. *The Improvement Guide: A Practical Approach to Enhancing Organizational Performance.* San Francisco: Jossey-Bass Publishers; 1996.

This book provides critical knowledge about improvement. It is the base upon which the work contained in this Guide was built.

Sahney VK. Managing variability in demand: A strategy for productivity improvement in health care services. *Health Care Manage Rev.* 1982(Spring):37–41.

This article provides a good discussion of demand management.

Shukla RK. Admissions monitoring and scheduling to improve work flow in hospitals. *Inquiry.* 1985;22:92–101.

Although this article addresses inpatient staffing and nurse productivity, and is relatively technical, it does contain concepts that are applicable to other areas as well.

Silva D. Capacity management: Get the level of detail right. *Hosp Mater Manage.* 1994;15(4):67–74.

A detailed discussion of capacity management.

U.S. Preventive Services Task Force. *Guide to Clinical Preventive Services.* 2nd ed. Baltimore: Williams & Wilkins; 1996.

This guide reports on over 200 commonly performed preventive practices.

AMBULATORY DELAYS, WAITING TIMES, AND ACCESS

Antle DW, Reid RA. Managing service capacity in an ambulatory care clinic. *Hosp Health Serv Adm.* 1988;33(2):201–211.

A framework with which to think about managing capacity.

Armstrong D, Britten N, Grace J. Measuring general practitioner referrals: Patient, workload and list size effects. *J R Coll Gen Pract.* 1988;38:494–497.

This analysis of predictors of general practitioner referrals to hospitals for additional outpatient care in the U.K.'s National Health Service examines provider utilization differences.

Bertera RL. The effects of workplace health promotion on absenteeism and employee costs in a large industrial population. *Am J Public Health.* 1990;80:1101–1105.

One of many articles that examines how workplace programs can lead to improved health and, therefore, reduced demand for healthcare services.

Connelly JE, Philbrick JT, Smith GR, Wymer A. Health perceptions of primary care patients and the influence on health care utilization. *Med Care.* 1989;27(3 Suppl):S99–S109.

Persons with low health perceptions in this study accounted for approximately 5% of office visits, suggesting the need for intervention in this group of patients.

Connelly JE, Smith GR, Philbrick JT, Kaiser DL. Healthy patients who perceive poor health and their use of primary care services. *J Gen Intern Med.* 1991;6:47–51.

This study suggests that 21% of adult primary care patients have health perceptions lower than expected for their levels of physical health and that these low perceptions correlate with increased utilization of resources.

Counte MA, Glandon GL. A panel study of life stress, social support, and the health services utilization of older persons. *Med Care.* 1991;29:348–361.

This complex psychosocial study links the combination of high life-stress exposure and low social support to increased rates of health services utilization.

Deguchi JJ, Inui TS, Martin DP. Measuring provider productivity in ambulatory care. *J Ambulatory Care Manage.* 1984;May:29–38.

The authors explore the use of a central scheduling system to improve the use of ambulatory physicians' time at a VA hospital.

Delio SA, Hein G. *The Making of an Efficient Physician.* Englewood, Colo.: Medical Group Management Association; 1995.

A very practical and readable book that describes the key aspects of building an effective and efficient office practice. It can be ordered by calling MGMA at (303) 799–1111.

Elsenhans VD, Marquardt C, Bledsoe T. Use of self-care manual shifts utilization pattern. *HMO Pract.* 1995;9(2):88–90.

Educating patients to provide appropriate self-care can significantly reduce demand for services.

Federa RD, Bilodeau TW. The productivity quest. *J Ambulatory Care Manage.* 1984;August:5–11.

A useful discussion that addresses the difficult topic of productivity.

Fries JF, Bloch DA, Harrington H, et al. Two-year results of a randomized controlled trial of a health promotion program in a retiree population: The Bank of America study. *Am J Med.* 1993;94:455–462.

Specific health promotion programs appropriately designed can both improve health risk status and reduce costs.

Golaszewski T, Snow D, Lynch W, et al. A benefit-to-cost analysis of a work-site health promotion program. *J Occup Med.* 1992;34:1164–1172.

This relatively technical study demonstrates the cost savings achieved by using health promotion programs even though these programs require up-front investments.

Goldberg HI, Cohen DI, Hershey CO. A randomized controlled trial of academic group practice. Improving the operation of the medicine clinic. *JAMA.* 1987; 257:2051–2055.

Adopting a group practice model improves clinic productivity, enhances patient flow, and decreases unscheduled clinic visits.

Hey M. Self-care, values lead to healthy communities. *Health Prog.* 1994;75:70–72, 79.

Self-care significantly cuts inappropriate utilization. This article describes a number of resources that can be used for self-care promotion.

Hodge RH, Gwin P, Mehl D. Productivity monitoring in ambulatory care settings. *J Ambulatory Care Manage.* 1985;8:28–35.

A relatively detailed discussion regarding ambulatory physician productivity; one of the few articles in the literature that addresses this topic.

Kemper DW. *Healthwise Handbook.* Boise, Idaho: Healthwise; 1995.
A widely used manual for self-care that can be used to manage demand for services. It may be ordered by calling Healthwise at (208) 345-1161.

Leigh JP, Fries JF. Health habits: Health care use and costs in a sample of retirees. *Inquiry.* 1992;29:44–54.
A study that examines how health habits of retirees affect their use of health services and subsequent cost. This study has implications for shaping demand for health services in this demographic group.

Lorig K, Kraines RG, Brown BW, Richardson N. A workplace health education program that reduces outpatient visits. *Med Care.* 1985;23:1044–1054.
Low cost, self-care workplace health intervention programs can significantly reduce outpatient visits. The techniques used in this study include workplace presentations, distribution of self-help books, and completion of self-administered questionnaires.

Lorig KR, Maxonson PD, Holman HR. Evidence suggesting that health education for self-management in patients with chronic arthritis has sustained health benefits while reducing healthcare costs. *Arthritis Rheum.* 1993;36:439–446.
Implementation of an Arthritis Self-Management Program produces significant reductions in pain, physician visits, and physical disability.

Lynam PF, Smith T, Dwyer J. Client flow analysis: A practical management technique for outpatient clinic settings. *Int J Qual Health Care.* 1994;6:179–186.
Client flow analysis is a method of examining patient flow through a clinic and optimizing use of providers' time.

Pelletier K. A review and analysis of the health and cost-effective outcome studies of comprehensive health promotion and disease prevention programs. *Am J Health Promot.* 1991;5:311–315.
A useful summary of studies that have examined health promotion and disease prevention programs.

Reid RA, Antle DW. Effective ambulatory service capacity management. *DRG Monit.* 1989;6(5):1–8.
The authors present a framework for ambulatory care capacity management including both demand-smoothing and supply-matching strategies.

Smith DM, Martin DK, Langefeld CD, et al. Primary care physician productivity: The physician factor. *J Gen Intern Med.* 1995;10:495–503.
Physician practice patterns rather than clinic or patient characteristics may account for most of the variation in physician productivity. Interventions to increase productivity need to consider methods to affect physician behavior.

Smoller M. Telephone calls and appointment requests. Predictability in an unpredictable world. *HMO Pract.* 1992;6(2):25–29.

A practical article providing a method for planning and effectively providing outpatient office appointments.

Tanner JL, Cockerham WC, Spaeth JL. Predicting medical utilization. *Med Care.* 1983;21:360–369.

This technical paper describes the use of a variable that measures the presence of symptoms as well as the person's own evaluation of the necessity for medical care for the symptoms experienced to predict physician utilization.

Tesch B, Lee H, McDonald M. Reducing the rate of missed appointments among patients new to a primary care clinic. *J Ambulatory Care Manage.* 1984;August:32–41.

This study demonstrates techniques that can reduce missed appointments by new patients using a flexible scheduling system.

Vickery DM, Fries JF. *Take Care of Yourself.* Reading, Mass.: Addison-Wesley; 1989.

A very usable self-care book developed by two of the leading experts in this field.

Vickery DM, Kalmer H, Lowty D, et al. The effect of a self-care education program on medical visits. *JAMA.* 1983;250:2952–2956.

This study estimates that decreased utilization associated with self-care educational interventions could result in a savings of approximately $2.50 to $3.50 for each dollar spent on the educational interventions.

Vickery DM, Lynch WD. Demand management: Enabling patients to use medical care appropriately. *J Occup Environ Med.* 1995;37:551–557.

A detailed discussion of the nature of healthcare demand as well as the management issues that address demand.

Vickery DN, Golaszewski TJ, Wright ED, Kalmer H. The effect of self-care interventions on the use of medical services within a Medicare population. *Med Care.* 1988;26:580–588.

Programs for education or home self-care can be used to reduce the demand for outpatient services while having no negative impact on the quality of health.

Who 'ya gonna call?: Telephonic demand management. *Market Pulse.* 1995;September:4–6.

A review of two national telephonic demand management companies.

EMERGENCY DEPARTMENT DELAYS AND WAITING TIMES

Bluth EI, Lambert DJ, Lohmann TP, et al. Improvement in 'stat' laboratory turnaround time. A model continuous quality improvement project. *Arch Intern Med.* 1992;152:837–840.

A quality improvement program that saved both time and money for this institution has implications for patient flow through emergency departments and urgent care settings.

Matson TA, McNamara P, eds. *The Hospital Emergency Department: A Guide to Operational Excellence.* Chicago, Ill.: American Hospital Publishing, Inc; 1992.

This book contains useful and innovative ideas for managing emergency departments and urgent care units.

Saunders CE, Makens PK, Leblanc LJ. Modeling emergency department operations using advanced computer simulation systems. *Ann Emerg Med.* 1989;18:134–140.

The authors develop a computer simulation model of emergency department operations and use it to predict the results of changes in the ED system.

Smeltzer CH, Curtis L. An analysis of emergency department time: Laying the groundwork for efficiency standards. *QRB.* 1987;13:240–242.

This and the following article by the same authors analyzes waiting times in EDs and suggests strategies for improving this process.

Smeltzer CH, Curtis L. Analyzing patient time in the emergency department. *QRB.* 1986;12:380–382.

Wait time plummets after hospital fast-tracks minor ED cases. *QI/TQM.* 1995;August:89–91.

This is a case study.

OPERATING ROOM DELAYS

Benchmarking helps hospital match hotel admission times. *QI/TQM.* 1994;January:10–11.

This is a case study: although benchmarking will not provide the knowledge necessary for change, it can serve to set goals for the organization and provide ideas for change.

'Best performers' work to keep surgeons happy. *OR Manager.* 1996;12(1):1,11–12.

This is a case study: flexible scheduling, data collection and utilization in decision making, and communication are important for running an efficient operating room.

Flexible staffing for OR's peaks and valleys. *OR Manager.* 1996;12(1):13,16.
This is a case study: a discussion about creative and flexible staffing to maximize efficiency.

Hospital-based same-day surgery center tunes up for race with freestanding center. *Hosp Benchmarks.* 1994;May:61–65.
This is a case study.

Information eases patient anxiety in the ED. *Hosp Benchmarks.* 1995;April:13–15.
This is a case study.

OR Manager. Boulder, Colo.: OR Manager, Inc.
This monthly newsletter of quality improvement ideas for managing operating rooms is recommended for all OR managers.

Prepare your OR now for a Stage 4 market. *OR Manager.* 1996;12(1):1,6–8.
This illustrates how organizations can use changes in the marketplace to stimulate improvements in their operating rooms.

Shukla RK, Ketcham JS, Ozcan YA. Comparison of subjective versus data-based approaches for improving efficiency of operating room scheduling. *Health Serv Manage Res.* 1990;3(2):74–81.
This study examines the best methods for estimating length of surgery for operating room scheduling systems.

Study identifies 'better performers' in the OR. *OR Manager.* 1995;11(9):1,6–8,10–12.
A January 1995 study by the University Hospital Consortium identifies best practices regarding key processes in the OR.

Study identifies best practices in ambulatory surgery centers. *OR Manager.* 1993;9(1):1,8–9.
This is a case study.